KETO COMFORT FOOD CLASSICS

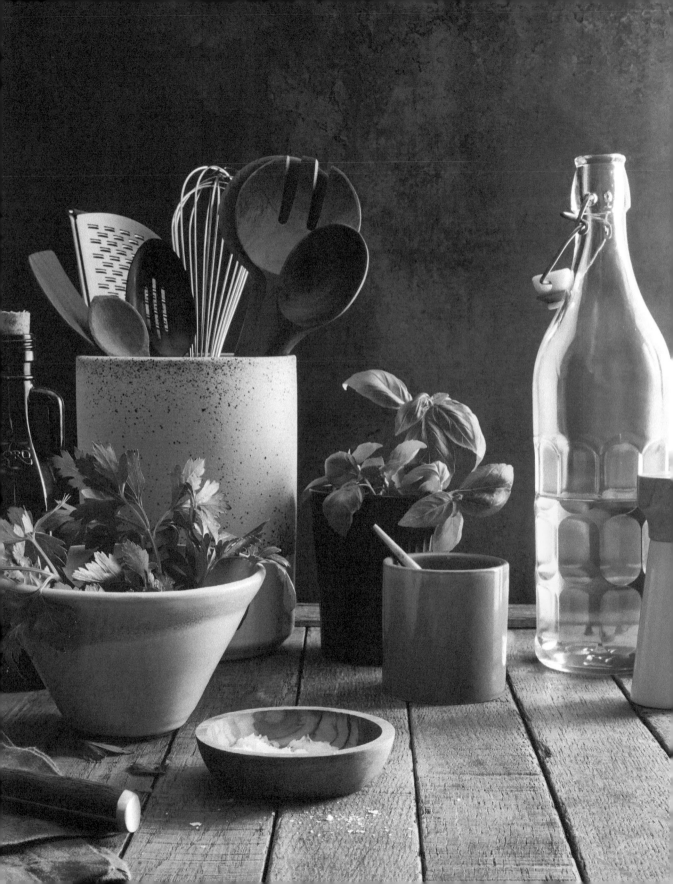

KETO COMFORT FOOD *Classics*

YOUR FAVORITE RECIPES MADE KETO

Kate Bay Jaramillo

Photography by Laura Flippen

ROCKRIDGE PRESS

For general information on our other products and services or to obtain technical support, please contact
our Customer Care Department within the United States at (866) 744-2665, or outside the United States at
(510) 253-0500.

Rockridge Press publishes its books in a variety of electronic and print formats. Some content that appears in
print may not be available in electronic books, and vice versa.

TRADEMARKS: Rockridge Press and the Rockridge Press logo are trademarks or registered trademarks of
Callisto Media Inc. and/or its affiliates, in the United States and other countries, and may not be used without
written permission. All other trademarks are the property of their respective owners. Rockridge Press is not
associated with any product or vendor mentioned in this book.

Interior and Cover Designer: Darren Samuel
Art Producer: Meg Baggott
Editor: Britt Bogan and Justin Hartung
Production Editor: Ruth Sakata Corley

Photography © 2020 Laura Flippen
Author photo courtesy of Samantha Tackeff

ISBN: Print 978-1-64739-715-9 | eBook 978-1-64739-716-6

R0

To Mario, Martina, Presley, Irie, and Madden.
Thank you for being my biggest source of support and inspiration,
and for being fearless recipe testers.

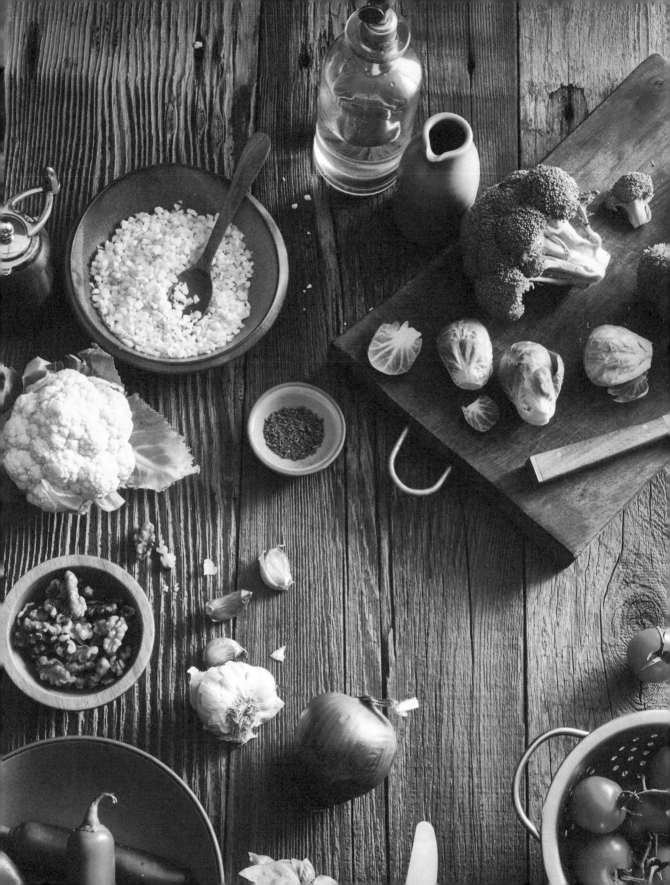

Contents

Introduction

"This is the strategy I use to help my clients lose the most amount of weight as quickly as possible." My ears perked up when I heard my nutrition instructor say these words. I had been working with a group of people who had plateaued in their weight loss for months. No matter how much they exercised or cut their calories, they just could not seem to lose another ounce.

As a fitness instructor and health coach, I felt I was failing my clients. When I learned about the ketogenic diet during this nutrition certification, I could see a way forward for these clients.

I took a deep dive into the ketogenic lifestyle, reading book after book, scouring the web for scholarly articles, and listening to every podcast I could find. Combining this knowledge with what I learned during my nutrition certification and my fitness instructor experience, I created an eight-week ketogenic lifestyle program.

Nine clients agreed to test my program, and six stayed with it for all eight weeks. Despite having been completely stalled for months, the average weight loss of the group was 20 pounds! Best of all, each person achieved levels of energy and mental clarity that they thought they had lost.

Since launching the Ketogenic Living Coach Certification, my little experiment has transformed thousands of lives all over the world.

I have always had a deep appreciation for food and love for cooking. I am a good instinctual cook, talented at combining flavors and ingredients to create delicious dishes. As a busy mom and business owner—and the primary cook for my family of six—I need to serve recipes my whole family will enjoy. There is no time to make multiple meals, so everyone in my house eats keto-friendly food.

My children are picky and honest and love a good meal, so I know that when they ask for more of one of my recipes, it has got to be tasty. The recipes in this cookbook have received their stamp of approval.

Transitioning from a standard American diet to a ketogenic lifestyle would not have been sustainable for me had I not reworked classic comfort foods into keto-friendly recipes. I am a true foodie and can't imagine a world without spaghetti and meatballs, grilled cheese, mac and cheese, and chocolate chip cookies.

Fortunately, I never have to. Neither do you.

In this book, you will find keto-fied recipes for classic comfort food dishes, made with easy-to-find ingredients. These are the recipes you'll reach for whenever you're feeling the need for a food equivalent of a warm hug.

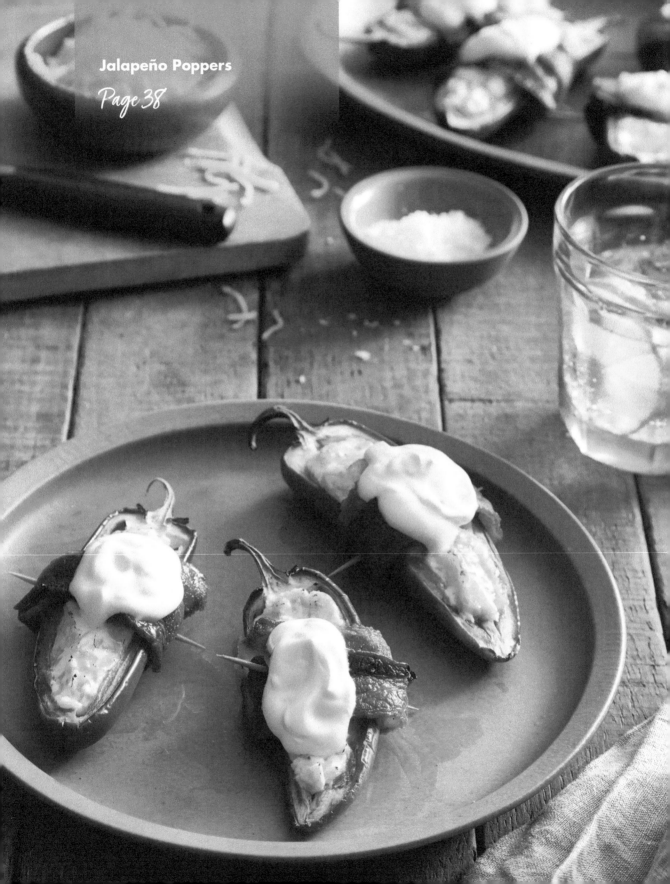

Jalapeño Poppers

Page 38

Chapter 1

GETTING COMFY WITH KETO

Transforming classic comfort food dishes into fat-fueled ketogenic treats is what this book is all about. All those delicious meals you may have crossed off your list when embarking on your ketogenic journey can now make their way back onto your plate.

Before we dive into the 100 crave-worthy keto-fied classic comfort food recipes, let's review the basic keto guidelines, including tips for stocking your kitchen and setting yourself up for success. This chapter covers how to track macros; foods to enjoy, limit, and avoid; staples and special ingredients; and essential kitchen equipment. Check out the 10 tips for keeping it keto, including how to cook for non-keto family members and what to do if you fall off the wagon.

This chapter details everything you need to get comfy and continue to enjoy your favorite foods.

Why Keto Works for Comfort Food

Even though we are serving up classic comfort food, the general rules of keto must still be followed to receive all the benefits of this fat-fueled lifestyle. Low carb, moderate protein, and lots of good healthy fats is the keto way, even—and especially—as it pertains to classic comfort food.

If you are new to keto, pay close attention to the Three Pillars of Keto (page 3). Even if you have been living *la vida* keto for a while now, the Pillars section ensures that we're on the same page.

Creamy, buttery, savory—comfort foods should feel like a warm hug from the inside. You can taste the love in each and every bite. Fortunately, many of those classic comfort food flavors and ingredients are staples in the ketogenic diet.

Keto embraces rich, healthy fats, such as butter and avocados. Dairy (including full-fat cheeses and heavy cream), beef, skin-on poultry, pork, eggs, and nuts appear in recipes throughout this book. If you grew up eating these foods, these recipes may remind you of happy, glowing times.

On the other hand, comfort foods can be synonymous with carb-heavy dishes, such as macaroni and cheese, spaghetti and meatballs, pizza, fried chicken, mashed potatoes, biscuits, brownies, cookies ... which don't jibe with keto. But fear not; classic comfort foods are well within your reach. As you will discover, the best cakes, pies, cookies, and custards can be keto-fied, as can breads, rice, and pastas.

Are you getting excited to jump in?

The Three Pillars of Keto

A ketogenic diet requires high amounts of fat, moderate amounts of protein, and low amounts of carbohydrates. These macronutrients (or macros for short) are the energy-giving components of food—the calories—that fuel the body. Grasping the concept of macros is important when adopting a keto lifestyle because you need to consume the right balance of fats, protein, and carbs to get into ketosis, stay in ketosis, and turn your body into a fat-burning machine.

How your body processes each macronutrient to reach and sustain ketosis can be determined through tracking your daily food intake. There are many free or low-cost apps that make macro tracking a cinch. If you're just beginning your keto journey, it's important to correctly enter all your food into the tracking app. For example, a serving size of almond butter might be a lot less than you imagined.

Macro tracking does not need to be complicated or done forever. Once you get an idea of how your body responds to certain foods, you will know whether to include them in your diet. Think of macro tracking as a tool to help you in the beginning of your journey or to use anytime you go off track or hit a plateau.

So, just how much of each macronutrient should you consume each day? The general ratio for a ketogenic diet is:

→ 70 to 75 percent calories from fat

→ 20 to 25 percent calories from protein

→ 5 to 10 percent calories from carbohydrates

LOW CARBOHYDRATE

A keto diet is low in carbohydrates. Did you know that carbs are the only nonessential macronutrient? This may sound crazy if you have ever been told to "carb up" for energy, but understand that through a process called gluconeogenesis, protein can be an energy source instead.

Carbs are made up of fiber, sugars, and starches. Because fiber is not fully digested, it has minimal impact on blood sugar levels. For this reason, many individuals following a ketogenic diet count net carbs, which can be calculated with this formula:

TOTAL CARBS – DIETARY FIBER – SUGAR ALCOHOLS (WHEN APPLICABLE) = NET CARBS

Fiber-rich and nutrient-dense carbohydrate sources such as broccoli, cauliflower, spinach, strawberries, and blackberries are best for keto comfort food dishes.

MODERATE PROTEIN

Protein is essential. Proteins are the building blocks of the body and play a vital role in almost all biological processes. Keto calls for moderate protein intake, which could mean anywhere from 0.6 to 1.1 grams of protein per pound of lean body weight (total weight – percent of body fat = lean body weight).

Beef burgers, chicken thighs, salmon, and eggs are wonderful sources of protein for ketogenic dieters.

Fat is also essential, required for energy, growth, development, vitamin absorption, organ health, and more. You may be wondering how you'll hit your daily fat intake, but it's actually very easy because fats provide 9 calories per gram (twice as much as proteins or carbs).

The best, most flavorful sources of fat to keep you fueled are butter, heavy cream, avocado, olive oil, coconut oil, coconut milk, and ghee.

TRACKING MACROS

Getting into and staying in ketosis means consuming the right macronutrient ratio. To make it easier for you to figure this out, there are several good macro tracking apps (see page 170 for recommendations). All you do is enter your meals and ensure that you stay within the ideal range of 70 to 75 percent fat, 20 to 25 percent protein, and 5 to 10 percent carbohydrates. As you get into a groove, macro tracking may simply become a tool to use occasionally when and if your goals change.

Tracking macros is also important because it can reveal "carb creep" — consuming more carbohydrates than you think. Measure your food and enter the amounts correctly.

Eat This, Not That

The next page lists foods to enjoy, limit, and avoid when stocking your keto kitchen. Keto emphasizes eating healthy fats and fresh, whole-food ingredients. Organic, grass-fed, pastured, and/or wild-caught protein sources are best. You'll see some keto-friendly foods in the "limit" category; this is because of their high carb count. Carbs and sugars hide in many processed foods, so look for foods in their most natural state and with as few ingredients as possible. Read the labels!

EAT THIS, NOT THAT

	ENJOY
DRINKS	water, sparkling water, flavored and unsweetened sparkling water, coffee and tea (both unsweetened or sweetened with a sugar-free keto-approved sweetener), unsweetened nut milks, unsweetened coconut milk
HERBS, VEGETABLES, AND FRUITS	asparagus, avocados, basil, broccoli, cauliflower, celery, collard greens, coriander, cucumber, cumin, green beans, lettuce, mushrooms, olives, parsley, radish, rosemary, sage, sauerkraut, spinach, Swiss chard, thyme, zucchini
GRAINS	N/A
DAIRY	butter, cream cheese, ghee, full-fat cheeses, heavy cream, whole-milk ricotta
NUTS AND SEEDS	N/A
FISH AND SHELLFISH	cod, crab, lobster, salmon, scallops, shrimp, tuna (canned, solid, in water or olive oil)
MEAT AND POULTRY	beef, bone broth, chicken, eggs, pork, turkey, sugar-free bacon, uncured sausage
OILS	avocado, MCT (< 320°F), olive, refined coconut, unrefined/virgin coconut
OTHER	apple cider vinegar, avocado oil-based mayonnaise
SPICES AND SEASONINGS	mustard, pure vanilla extract, sea salt
SWEETENERS	Lakanto Maple Flavored Syrup, liquid stevia, monk fruit, erythritol

LIMIT	AVOID
spirits (bourbon, brandy, gin, rum, tequila, vodka, whisky), unsweetened tea, wine (dry red, dry white)	beer, cocktails, sweetened coffee, energy drinks, fruit juices, lemonade, sodas, wine (sweet red, sweet white)
blackberries, blueberries, Brussels sprouts, garlic, kale, lemon, lime, onion, oregano, peppers, raspberries, strawberries, tomatoes	apples, bananas, beans, beets, butternut squash, carrots, dried fruits, grapes, legumes, lentils, mangos, nectarines, oranges, peaches, pears, peas, pineapple, potatoes, yams
N/A	barley, bread, breaded animal products (meats, poultry, and seafood), buckwheat, cereal, corn, crackers, millet, oats, pasta, popcorn, pretzels, quinoa, rice, sandwich wraps, wheat, whole grains
N/A	fat-free and low-fat dairy products, milk (cow, goat, sheep, etc.)
almonds, Brazil nuts, hazelnuts, macadamia nuts, pecans, sunflower seeds, walnuts	cashews
N/A	N/A
minimally processed/uncured lunch meats, pork rinds, uncured hot dogs	processed deli meats, bacon with added sugar, flavored rotisserie chicken with added sugar, breaded meats and poultry, meats and poultry covered in sugary sauces (barbecue, many Chinese sauces)
N/A	canola, corn, cottonseed, peanut, safflower, sesame, soybean, sunflower, vegetable
almond flour, chocolate chips (sugar free), chocolate (dark 85%+), coconut cream, coconut flour, coconut milk (full fat), ketchup (sugar free)	margarine, vegetable shortening
garlic powder, chili powder, cinnamon, onion powder, paprika	N/A
xylitol	agave syrup, aspartame, brown rice syrup, brown sugar, coconut sugar, dextrose, fructose, high-fructose corn syrup, honey, maltitol, maltodextrin, maple syrup, molasses, saccharin, sucralose, sugar

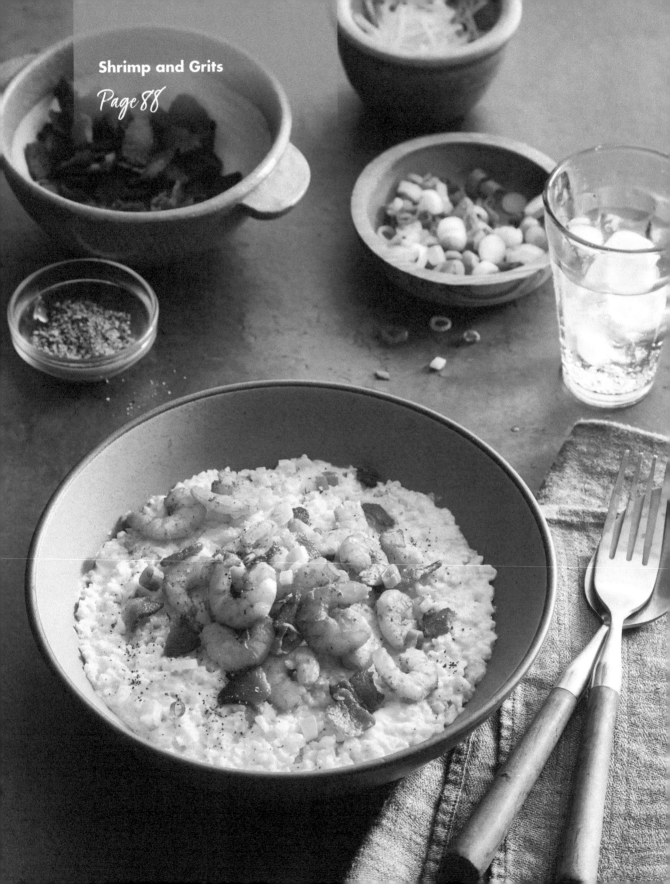

Shrimp and Grits

Page 88

A word about fats: Even healthy fats can become unhealthy when they exceed their smoke point—the point at which a fat will smoke, burn, and begin to release free radicals, which are associated with many chronic and even life-threatening diseases. When you want to cook at high heat, choose oils with a high smoke point:

Avocado oil: 520°F

Ghee: 485°F

Olive oil (virgin): 420°F

Olive oil (extra virgin): 400°F

Coconut oil (refined): 400°F

Coconut oil (unrefined): 350°F

Butter: 350°F

The Keto Comfort Kitchen

Stocking up on the foods mentioned here will set you up for preparing the classic comfort food recipes in this book so that whenever you get a craving for something nurturing and delicious, you'll be good to go.

STAPLES AND SPECIAL INGREDIENTS

You'll want to keep these essentials on hand to easily whip up a dish. Pick up an unsweetened nut milk of your choice and a jar of cream of tartar, too.

FLOUR REPLACEMENT

Use fine almond flour (the more coarsely ground almond meal has a mealier texture). For nut allergies, substitute sunflower seed flour or coconut flour. When purchasing, check the ingredients to make sure the only thing listed is almonds, sunflower seeds, or coconut.

NUT OR SEED BUTTER

Use almond butter; it should only have one or two ingredients: almonds and sea salt. For nut allergies, substitute sunflower seed butter.

COCONUT OIL

This keto staple comes in two varieties. Refined (also called virgin or extra virgin) is processed in a way that removes the coconut smell and flavor. (Avoid partially hydrogenated refined coconut oil; it's highly processed and contains trans fats.) Unrefined retains the coconut flavor and has a lower smoke point than refined.

Choosing between refined and unrefined comes down to flavor preference and how you will be using the oil. (See page 9 for their smoke points.)

PORK RINDS

Pork rinds contain zero carbohydrates and moderate amounts of protein and are high in fat. Basic pork rinds are a great alternative to bread crumbs; just crush them. Pork cracklins make a great keto-friendly snack. Avoid flavored pork rinds, as many contain artificial ingredients and sugars.

SHIRATAKI NOODLES AND MIRACLE RICE

Shirataki noodles and miracle rice are zero-carb. They are made almost entirely of water, held together with glucomannan fiber from the konjac root. Rinsing and drying them before cooking gives them a texture more similar to traditional pastas and rice.

MASCARPONE

This soft, buttery Italian cream cheese contains twice the fat of regular cream cheese and adds smooth, rich texture to recipes. Mascarpone is sweeter than cream cheese, but without any added sugar.

SUGAR-FREE SWEET THINGS

Erythritol: This sugar alcohol is a popular keto sugar substitute. Erythritol is not fully digested and therefore has minimal impact on blood sugar. It can be used 1:1 as a sugar substitute in most recipes.

Chocolate: Choose sugar-free chocolate chips, such as Lily's or ChocZero. ChocZero is soy-free.

Pure flavor extracts and oils: These are an excellent way to add taste without the carbohydrates. Craft stores such as Michael's are a good place to find flavored oils.

MCT OIL

Medium-chain triglycerides (MCTs) are the same type of saturated fat found in coconut oil. The advantage of MCT is that it travels straight to the liver and gets used immediately for energy or turned into ketones. Bulletproof Brain Octane is my go-to brand. MCT oil can be purchased in powder, pill, and liquid form.

ESSENTIAL EQUIPMENT

Having the right tools for the job is just as important as the ingredients. You may already have these in your kitchen; if not, consider getting them as you will use them to create keto comfort food dishes that taste just like the "real thing."

→ Baking dish

→ Baking sheets

→ Cheese grater

→ Electric hand or stand mixer

→ Loaf pan

→ Parchment paper

→ Roasting pan

→ Vegetable spiralizer

→ Whisk

OTHER SWEETENERS

In addition to erythritol, some recipes in this book call for two different sweeteners: Sukrin Gold and Lakanto Maple Flavored Syrup. Both can be ordered online.

Traditional baking recipes often call for white or brown sugar. Although sometimes used interchangeably, the two taste noticeably different. The same goes for erythritol and Sukrin Gold. Sukrin Gold adds a molasses-like richness. Certain brown sugar substitutes, such as golden monk fruit, have a very strong cooling effect in the mouth. Because Sukrin Gold contains both erythritol and stevia, the mouthfeel is more like regular brown sugar.

Many sugar-free syrups contain artificial sweeteners that can cause a spike in blood sugar, kicking the body out of ketosis. Lakanto Maple Flavored Syrup is made with monk fruit, a natural sugar that has no impact on blood sugar. Although it is a bit thinner in consistency, it tastes just like regular maple syrup.

10 Tips for Keeping It Keto

Making any kind of change may feel daunting at first, but the longer you follow a ketogenic diet, the more confident you will become in your ability to make this lifestyle stick. Here are 10 tips to keep calm and keto on:

1. **Track macros.** Track your macros (see page 170 for apps).

2. **Ditch non-keto foods.** Update your kitchen staples and prioritize whole, nutrient-dense foods (see page 6).

3. **Read labels.** Ingredients are listed from the highest percentage to the lowest; the first ingredient should be a whole food.

4. **Cooking for non-keto people.** Keep things simple. Choose fattier cuts of protein and low-carb vegetables. Berries for dessert. Rice or gluten-free pasta on standby. Gluten can be inflammatory, so it's best to avoid it when possible.

5. **Plan meals ahead.** Take inventory of what you already have, make a list, and only purchase what's on it.

6. **Cook at home.** I've got you covered with the recipes in this book!

7. **Keep keto when eating out.** Check out the restaurant's menu in advance and plan to order a non-breaded piece of protein and low-carb veggies. Drink water. Avoid the bread basket.

8. **Drink water.** It is easy to mistake hunger for thirst. Aim to drink half your body weight in ounces per day.

9. **Practice mindful eating.** Focus on chewing and enjoying every tasty bite. You will feel fuller faster and will stay within your macronutrient goals.

10. **Weather accidents.** Sometimes you will consume grains, gluten, or sugar. Is this the end of the world? Absolutely not! Don't beat yourself up; turn to these comfort food recipes and jump back into ketosis.

About the Recipes

Comfort foods can evoke any number of feelings, such as reviving happy memories or bringing a smile to your face while warming your belly. This cookbook's recipes have been selected because they are classic comfort food dishes, well-known treasures loved by just about everyone.

Adapting the most classic comfort food dishes to fit a ketogenic lifestyle is an easy process that results in meals you will make over and over again. Giving these classics a ketogenic update allows you to eat your way to optimal health.

To make it as simple as possible for you to recreate these comfort food dishes in your own home, most recipes in this book can be prepared using 10 ingredients or fewer (not counting salt, pepper, butter, or oil).

Because tracking macros is a tool that enhances your chances of success with the ketogenic diet, all the recipes include macro percentages and complete nutritional information, making them easy to plug into your tracking app and keep on ketoing on.

Now, let's get cooking!

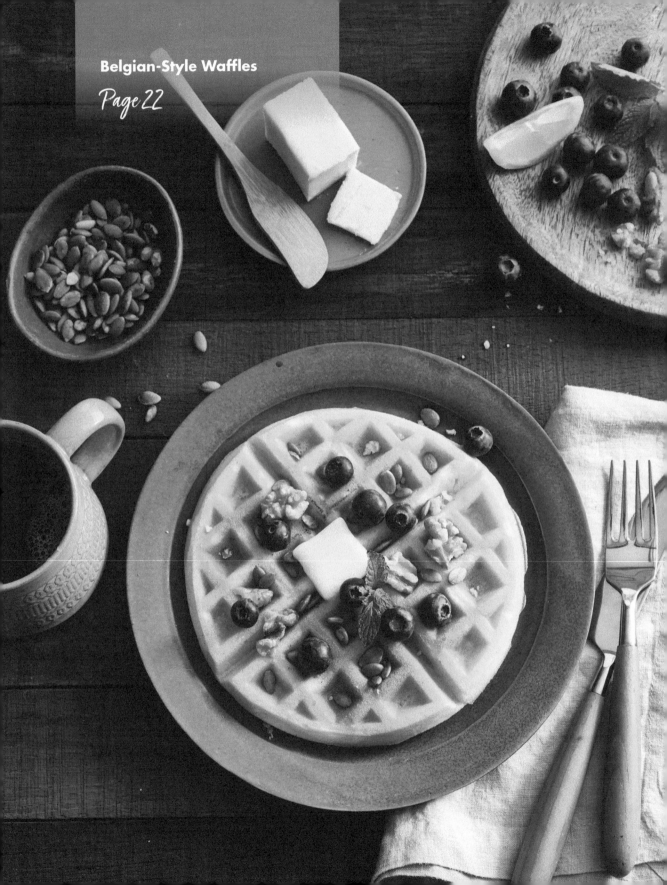

Belgian-Style Waffles

Page 22

Chapter 2

BREAKFAST

Butter Biscuits and Sausage Gravy

SERVES 4 | PREP TIME: 40 MINUTES | COOK TIME: 10 MINUTES

Close your eyes. Imagine breathing in the aroma of freshly baked biscuits ready to be covered in rich, creamy sausage gravy. Traditional biscuits are not in the slightest bit keto-friendly, but by subbing out the carb-heavy flour, these butter biscuits are your comfort food breakfast fix.

FOR THE BISCUITS

12 tablespoons (1½ sticks) frozen salted butter
3 cups fine almond flour
¼ cup coconut flour, plus more for dusting
2 teaspoons baking powder
3 tablespoons erythritol
1 cold egg, whisked
1 cup cold heavy cream
1½ tablespoons melted butter (optional)

FOR THE SAUSAGE GRAVY

½ pound pork breakfast sausage
4 ounces cream cheese, at room temperature
½ cup heavy cream
½ cup beef broth
Pinch nutmeg
¼ teaspoon garlic powder
½ teaspoon freshly ground black pepper

Per Serving (1 biscuit with ½ cup sausage gravy): Calories: 1,388; Total fat: 134g; Total carbs: 34g; Fiber: 12g; Net carbs: 22g; Protein: 33g; Macronutrients: Fat: 84%; Protein: 9%; Carbs: 7%

TO MAKE THE BISCUITS

1. Preheat the oven to 450°F. Line a baking sheet with parchment paper.
2. Grate the butter into tiny pieces and return to the freezer for 10 to 15 minutes.
3. In a large bowl, whisk the almond and coconut flours, baking powder, and erythritol together. Add the butter and use a spoon to stir until incorporated. Stir in the egg and cream.
4. Sprinkle some coconut flour on your work surface and your hands. Pat the dough to a ¾-inch thickness. Using a round dough cutter or the top of a glass, cut the dough into 12 to 14 circles. Press the scraps together to cut more circles. Sprinkle with coconut flour if the dough becomes too sticky.
5. Place the biscuits on the prepared baking sheet. Brush with melted butter (if using).
6. Bake for 10 to 12 minutes, until golden on top and a toothpick comes out clean.

TO MAKE THE SAUSAGE GRAVY

7. While the biscuits are baking, in a large saucepan over medium heat, cook the sausage, breaking it into small pieces with the back of the spoon, until browned, about 5 minutes. Drain the fat.

8. Return the pan to medium heat and stir in the cream cheese, cream, broth, nutmeg, garlic powder, and pepper.

9. Simmer, stirring frequently, until the sausage is cooked through and the liquid has thickened, about 8 minutes.

10. To serve, slice 4 biscuits in half and spoon the sausage gravy on top. Refrigerate leftovers for up to 3 days. The extra biscuits can be stored in an airtight container on the counter for up to two days, or frozen for up to one month. If frozen, they need to thaw completely before being warmed in the microwave for 30 seconds, or in the oven at 350°F for 2 to 3 minutes.

> **PREPARATION TIP:** Use a food processor to make the biscuits. Blitz the ice-cold butter and then pop it back in the freezer. Combine the dry ingredients in the food processor and then pulse in the butter until the dough is crumbly. Add the egg and cream and pulse again until it forms a dough. Follow the remaining instructions from there.

Classic Bacon and Eggs

SERVES 2 | PREP TIME: 5 MINUTES | COOK TIME: 15 MINUTES

A staple on every hometown diner menu—and in just about every keto diet—is the dynamic duo: bacon and eggs. Baking the bacon is a game-changer in taste, crispiness, and cleanup. Serve your eggs any way you like. The techniques provided here are my favorites for hitting the comfort food spot.

6 slices sugar-free bacon
2 tablespoons butter
4 eggs
Freshly ground black
  pepper (optional)

Per Serving (3 slices bacon and 2 eggs): Calories: 328; Total fat: 27g; Total carbs: 1g; Fiber: 0g; Net carbs: 1g; Protein: 20g; Macronutrients: Fat: 73%; Protein: 26%; Carbs: 1%

1. Preheat the oven to 350°F. Line a rimmed baking sheet with parchment paper. Line a plate with paper towels.

2. Place the bacon slices in a single layer, not overlapping, on the prepared baking sheet.

3. Bake for 13 to 17 minutes or until cooked the way you like it. Transfer to the prepared plate.

4. While the bacon is baking, in a medium frying pan over medium heat, melt the butter, swirling to coat the pan completely.

5. Crack each egg into a measuring cup or bowl and then slowly pour into the pan.

6. Allow the eggs to cook undisturbed for about 2 minutes, just until the whites are set.

7. Slide a spatula under each egg and gently flip. Cook for another 1 to 2 minutes (shorter for a runny yolk, longer for a harder one).

8. Season with pepper (if using) and serve with the bacon.

Ricotta Pancakes

SERVES 4 | PREP TIME: 5 MINUTES | COOK TIME: 20 MINUTES

Soft and fluffy, short stack or tall, the pancake is perhaps the most comforting breakfast food of all. Here, we swap out traditional buttermilk for keto-friendly whole-milk ricotta cheese. The ricotta adds an almost custard-like texture that allows these pancakes to live up to their name: truly a cake made in a pan. Top with butter, sugar-free maple syrup, sugar-free chocolate chips, whipped cream, fresh berries—you really can't go wrong.

5 ounces whole-milk ricotta cheese, drained
⅓ cup granular erythritol
2 teaspoons vanilla extract
2 tablespoons unsweetened vanilla almond milk
1 cup almond flour
1 teaspoon baking powder
⅛ teaspoon cream of tartar
4 large eggs
4 tablespoons butter, divided

Per Serving (1 pancake):
Calories: 401; Total fat: 35g;
Total carbs: 25g; Fiber: 3g;
Sugar alcohol: 16g;
Net carbs: 6g; Protein: 15g;
Macronutrients: Fat: 75%;
Protein: 15%; Carbs: 10%

1. Preheat the oven to its lowest setting. Place a baking sheet in the oven.
2. In a large bowl, whisk together the ricotta, erythritol, vanilla, almond milk, almond flour, baking powder, cream of tartar, and eggs until smooth. Thin the batter with almond milk if necessary.
3. In a small nonstick frying pan over medium-low heat, melt 1 tablespoon of butter.
4. Pour ¼ cup of batter into the pan and cook until golden, about 4 minutes per side.
5. Transfer the pancake to the baking sheet in the oven.
6. Repeat steps 3 to 5 until the batter has been used. Serve the pancakes with your favorite toppings. Refrigerate leftovers for up to 3 days or freeze for up to 1 month.

SUBSTITUTION TIP: Ditch the vanilla and kick it up a notch with 2 teaspoons of lemon zest. Replace the almond milk with 2 tablespoons of lemon juice.

Belgian-Style Waffles

MAKES 4 | PREP TIME: 5 MINUTES | COOK TIME: 10 MINUTES

A waffle station is a sign of a great breakfast buffet for me. However, traditional waffles are loaded with gluten and sugar, two ingredients that can kick your body out of ketosis. Fear not: These waffles come together even faster than the frozen kind and will keep your body in prime fat-burning mode.

4 large eggs

4 ounces full-fat cream cheese, at room temperature

1 tablespoon melted butter

1 teaspoon vanilla extract

½ teaspoon maple extract (optional)

¼ cup fine almond flour

1 tablespoon coconut flour

½ tablespoon baking powder

2 tablespoons granular erythritol

Pinch sea salt

1 tablespoon unsweetened almond milk (optional)

Coconut cooking spray or butter, for greasing

Per Serving (1 waffle):
Calories: 237; Total fat: 20g; Total carbs: 11g; Fiber: 1g; Sugar alcohol: 6g; Net carbs: 4g; Protein: 10g; Macronutrients: Fat: 74%; Protein: 17%; Carbs: 9%

1. Heat a waffle iron.
2. Put the eggs, cream cheese, butter, vanilla, maple extract (if using), almond and coconut flours, baking powder, erythritol, and salt in a blender in the order listed and blend on high speed until completely combined. Add the almond milk if you desire a thinner consistency and blend again until combined.
3. Spray the waffle iron with cooking spray.
4. Pour ¼ cup of batter onto the waffle iron and cook for 2 to 3 minutes or until browned and slightly crisped on both sides.
5. Remove the waffle. Repeat steps 3 and 4 to make 3 more waffles.
6. Serve with your favorite toppings. Refrigerate leftovers for up to 3 days or freeze for up to 1 month.

SUBSTITUTION TIP: Get creative with flavor extracts and toppings, as long as you keep them low-carb and keto-friendly. You may want to try banana extract and walnuts, apple extract and a pinch of cinnamon, or lemon extract with blueberries.

Banana Nut Muffins

MAKES 12 | PREP TIME: 10 MINUTES | COOK TIME: 25 MINUTES

Because bananas are a high-sugar fruit, they are left off a keto menu. But these muffins swap the actual fruit for banana extract, imparting all the flavor without additional carbs or sugar.

2½ cups fine almond flour
½ teaspoon baking soda
¼ teaspoon sea salt
1 teaspoon ground cinnamon
1½ teaspoons banana extract
2 large eggs, at room temperature
4 ounces full-fat sour cream
½ cup sugar-free maple syrup, plus 2 tablespoons, divided
⅓ cup chopped walnuts, plus 2 tablespoons, divided
1 tablespoon melted butter

Per Serving (1 muffin):
Calories: 224; Total fat: 18g; Total carbs: 12g; Fiber: 8g; Net carbs: 4g; Protein: 7g; Macronutrients: Fat: 69%; Protein: 11%; Carbs: 20%

1. Preheat the oven to 325°F. Line a 12-cup muffin tin with cupcake liners.
2. In a large bowl, whisk together the almond flour, baking soda, salt, and cinnamon.
3. In another large bowl, use an electric mixer (or spoon) to combine the banana extract, eggs, sour cream, and ½ cup of syrup.
4. Slowly pour the banana mixture into the almond flour mixture and thoroughly combine. Fold in ⅓ cup of walnuts.
5. Divide the muffin mixture evenly among the muffin cups. Bake for 20 to 25 minutes, until a toothpick inserted into a muffin center comes out clean. Transfer to a wire rack to cool.
6. In a small bowl, whisk together the remaining 2 tablespoons of syrup, 2 tablespoons of walnuts, and the melted butter.
7. When the muffins are cool enough to handle, spoon the walnut mixture evenly on top of each muffin and serve immediately. Refrigerate leftovers for up to 5 days or freeze for up to 2 months.

Denver Omelet Breakfast Bake

SERVES 6 | PREP TIME: 15 MINUTES | COOK TIME: 40 MINUTES

What better way to fuel your day than with a delicious Denver omelet? An omelet is a classic breakfast, but the carbs in onions and peppers can add up. This recipe reduces the vegetables and replaces them with a little extra protein. An easy one to meal prep and store, this dish provides a perfect ratio of keto macros.

Cooking spray
1 tablespoon olive oil
¼ cup diced white onion
½ large green bell
  pepper, diced
Sea salt
Freshly ground
  black pepper
10 large eggs
½ cup heavy cream
Pinch nutmeg (optional)
1½ cups cooked cubed ham
1 cup shredded cheddar
  cheese, divided

Per Serving: Calories: 343; Total fat: 26g; Total carbs: 5g; Fiber: <1g; Net carbs: 5g; Protein: 23g; Macronutrients: Fat: 68%; Protein: 27%; Carbs: 5%

1. Preheat the oven to 400°F. Spray a casserole dish with cooking spray.
2. In a small saucepan over medium heat, heat the olive oil. Add the onion and cook, stirring frequently, for 3 minutes or until soft and translucent.
3. Add the bell pepper and season with salt and pepper to taste. Cook for another 2 minutes, stirring, and then set aside.
4. In a large bowl, whisk together the eggs, cream, and nutmeg (if using) until well combined. Stir in the onion, pepper, ham, and ¾ cup of cheese.
5. Pour the omelet mixture into the prepared casserole dish. Top with remaining ¼ cup of cheese.
6. Bake for 30 to 35 minutes or until a toothpick inserted in the center comes out clean. Serve immediately or refrigerate for up to 5 days.

French Toast

SERVES 2 | PREP TIME: 10 MINUTES PLUS OVERNIGHT | COOK TIME: 5 MINUTES

Thick slices of bread, crispy on the outside and custardy on the inside, French toast is a filling and decadent breakfast. This recipe calls for day-old 90-Second Bread because it holds its texture in the cream and egg mixture. Fresh 90-Second Bread will taste great but may fall apart while cooking. Fresh berries and a sprinkle of powdered erythritol on top look beautiful.

2 batches 90-Second Bread (page 158; see Note)
2 large eggs
½ cup heavy cream
2 teaspoons erythritol
¼ teaspoon ground cinnamon
¼ teaspoon vanilla extract
2 tablespoons butter
Sugar-free maple syrup, for serving (optional)

Per Serving (2 slices): Calories: 684; Total fat: 66g; Total carbs: 12g; Fiber: 3g; Net carbs: 9g; Protein: 19g; Macronutrients: Fat: 85%; Protein: 11%; Carbs: 4%

1. Make the 90-Second Bread. Cool and store in an airtight container overnight.
2. In the morning, slice the bread in half.
3. In a medium bowl, whisk together the eggs, cream, erythritol, cinnamon, and vanilla.
4. Melt the butter in a small skillet over medium heat.
5. Dredge each slice of bread in the egg and cream mixture and place it in the skillet. Fry each slice until crispy, 2 to 3 minutes per side.
6. Transfer to a plate and drizzle with sugar-free syrup (if using).

NOTE: Make 90-Second Bread with 1 tablespoon coconut oil in lieu of the butter, plus ⅛ teaspoon cinnamon and ¼ teaspoon of erythritol added to the batter.

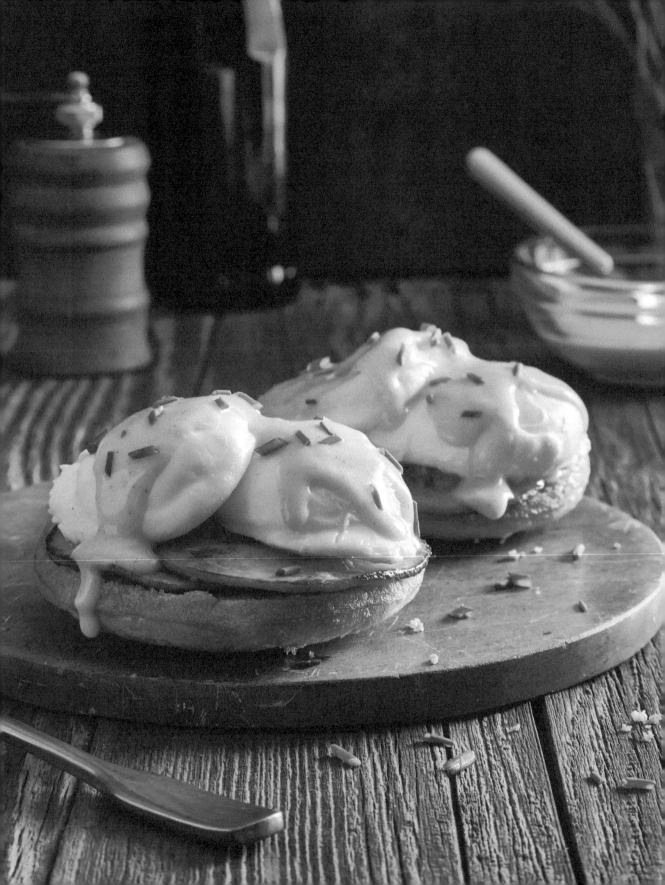

Easy Eggs Benedict

SERVES 4 | PREP TIME: 15 MINUTES | COOK TIME: 25 MINUTES

Eggs Benedict is my husband's favorite breakfast dish ever. Buttery hollandaise sauce covering a perfectly runny egg, nesting on a toasted English muffin, eggs Benedict is truly a treat for the taste buds. This keto version uses the simple 90-Second Bread and a blender hollandaise sauce.

8 slices Canadian bacon
4 batches 90-Second Bread
    (page 158; see Note)
1 tablespoon white vinegar
8 large eggs, plus 3 large
    egg yolks, divided
1 tablespoon freshly
    squeezed lemon juice
⅛ teaspoon paprika
10 tablespoons melted
    salted butter

Per Serving: Calories: 852; Total fat: 75g; Total carbs: 8g; Fiber: 2g; Net carbs: 6g; Protein: 40g; Macronutrients: Fat: 77%; Protein: 19%; Carbs: 4%

1. Preheat the oven to 325°F. Line a baking sheet with parchment paper.
2. Place the bacon in an even layer on the baking sheet. Bake for 10 minutes, flip, and bake for another 10 minutes. Remove from the oven and set aside.
3. While the bacon is baking, make the 90-Second Bread. When each piece is cool enough to handle, slice in half and toast.
4. Bring a large pot of water to a boil over high heat and then reduce the heat to low. Stir in the vinegar.
5. Working with one egg at a time, crack it onto a small plate, allowing the runny white to separate from the solid white surrounding the yolk. Gently pour the egg into the water. Multiple eggs can cook together, but you want to pour them in individually.
6. Set a timer for 3 minutes. When the eggs are done, remove them from the water with a slotted spoon.

> **NOTE:** Make 90-Second Bread with 1 tablespoon olive oil in lieu of the butter.

CONTINUED

7. While the eggs cook, combine the egg yolks, lemon juice, and paprika in a blender and blend on high speed for about 30 seconds.

8. Reduce the blender speed to its lowest setting. Drizzle in the melted butter and continue to blend for another 30 seconds or until completely incorporated.

9. To serve, top each toast slice with 2 bacon slices, 2 eggs, and one-fourth of the hollandaise.

SUBSTITUTION TIP: Replace the bacon with 4 cups of spinach sautéed in 2 tablespoons of olive oil for 3 to 5 minutes.

Granola Cereal

SERVES 8 | PREP TIME: 5 MINUTES | COOK TIME: 25 MINUTES

Traditional granola is made with oats and some form of sugar. If you have been missing granola's crunch, the coconut flakes, nuts, and chocolate chips in this recipe will provide the healthy, fat-fueled comfort fix you've been craving.

¼ cup creamy almond butter

2 tablespoons melted coconut oil

2 tablespoons sugar-free maple syrup

1 egg white

½ teaspoon vanilla extract

¼ teaspoon ground cinnamon

¾ cup unsweetened coconut flakes

¾ cup almond slivers

⅓ cup chopped pecans

2 tablespoons sugar-free chocolate chips

¼ teaspoon sea salt

Unsweetened nut milk, for serving

Per Serving (¼ cup): Calories: 241; Total fat: 22g; Total carbs: 9g; Fiber: 5g; Net carbs: 4g; Protein: 5g; Macronutrients: Fat: 77%; Protein: 8%; Carbs: 15%

1. Preheat the oven to 300°F. Line a rimmed baking sheet with parchment paper.
2. In a large bowl, whisk together the almond butter, coconut oil, maple syrup, egg white, and vanilla until well combined. Sprinkle in the cinnamon and whisk again.
3. Stir in the coconut flakes, almonds, pecans, and chocolate chips.
4. Spread the mixture in an even layer on the prepared baking sheet. Sprinkle evenly with the salt.
5. Bake for 10 to 12 minutes, rotate the baking sheet without stirring the granola, and bake for another 10 to 12 minutes. Watch carefully so the granola does not burn. It is done when the top browns.
6. Remove the baking sheet from the oven and allow the granola to cool completely.
7. Once cool, break the granola into clusters and store in an airtight container for up to 10 days. To enjoy immediately, place a serving of granola in a bowl and pour the nut milk over top.

SUBSTITUTION TIP: By swapping the almond butter for pumpkin puree, the cinnamon for pumpkin pie spice, and pumpkin seeds for the chocolate chips, you can enjoy a Pumpkin Spice Granola Cereal.

Jelly Donuts

MAKES 6 | PREP TIME: 15 MINUTES | COOK TIME: 15 MINUTES

Donuts were always a special treat my family reserved for a weekend morning. Pillowy soft, deep fried, and doused in sugar—so many things to find alluring! Because we use almond flour, these jelly donuts are denser in weight and texture than traditional donuts. If you prefer a glazed donut, simply mix ⅓ cup of powdered erythritol with 2 teaspoons of unsweetened vanilla almond milk.

Cooking spray
1 cup chopped ripe
   strawberries
⅓ cup water
1 envelope (¼ ounce)
   unflavored gelatin
½ cup erythritol, divided,
   plus 1 tablespoon
1 cup plus 2 tablespoons
   almond flour
½ teaspoon baking powder
2 large eggs
½ teaspoon apple
   cider vinegar
2 tablespoons unsweetened
   vanilla almond milk
2 tablespoons
   melted butter

Per Serving (1 donut): Calories: 193; Total fat: 16g; Total carbs: 24g; Fiber: 3g; Sugar alcohol: 18g; Net carbs: 3g; Protein: 8g; Macronutrients: Fat: 72%; Protein: 15%; Carbs: 13%

1. Preheat the oven to 350°F. Spray 6 cups of a muffin tin with cooking spray.
2. Puree the strawberries in a blender.
3. Pour the water into a medium saucepan over medium heat. Sprinkle the gelatin on top and then add ¼ cup of erythritol. Whisk for 2 to 3 minutes until completely combined.
4. Slowly whisk in the strawberries and allow the mixture to bubble. Turn the heat to low and cook, stirring occasionally, for 5 to 7 minutes until the puree has thickened. Remove from the heat and refrigerate to cool.
5. In a large bowl, mix together the almond flour, ¼ cup of erythritol, and the baking powder. Add the eggs, vinegar, and almond milk and mix into a thick dough.
6. Divide the dough into 6 equal pieces and drop into the prepared muffin cups. Bake in the center of the oven for 12 to 15 minutes or until lightly golden on top.

7. While the donuts bake, pour the strawberry jelly into a resealable plastic bag and cut off one of the corners. Pour the remaining 2 tablespoons of erythritol onto a small plate.

8. Once the donuts are cooked, remove them from the muffin tin, pour the butter all over them, and roll each donut in the erythritol.

9. Cut a deep slit into the side of each donut (not all the way through). Pipe strawberry jelly into each one. Serve immediately or store in an airtight container at room temperature for 1 more day.

> **MAKE AHEAD:** The jelly can be refrigerated for up to 7 days. When you are ready to use it, let it sit at room temperature while the donuts are baking.

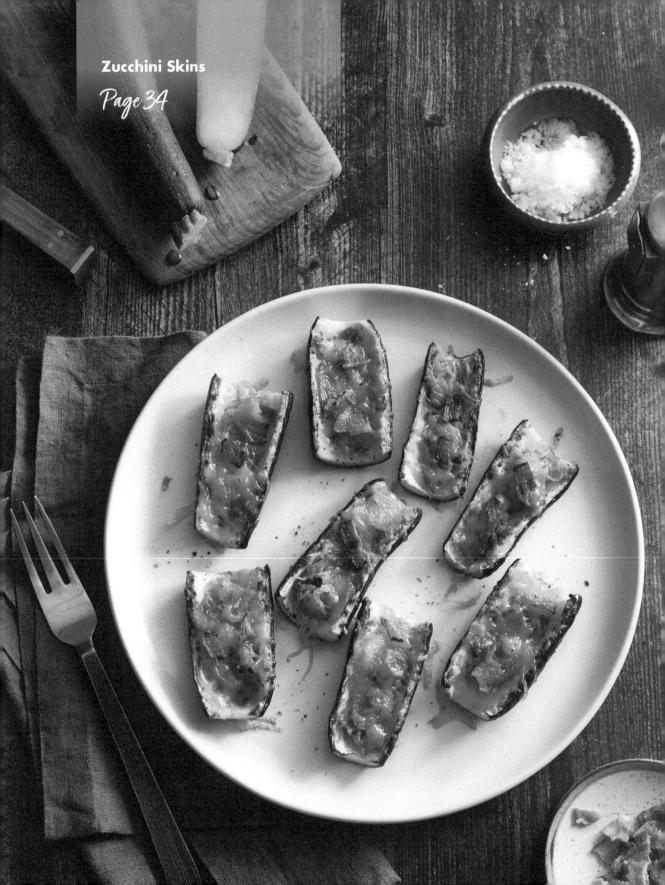

Zucchini Skins

Page 34

Chapter 3

SOUPS, SALADS, AND HANDHELDS

Zucchini Skins

Potatoes are a no-go for keto people, but zucchini makes an excellent replacement. They are sturdy enough to hold a mix of toppings and have a neutral flavor that allows each topping to shine. This method of cooking yields crispy zucchini skins that can't wait to be loaded up with your favorite fixin's.

2 medium zucchini, ends trimmed

2 teaspoons avocado oil, divided

4 slices bacon

¼ teaspoon sea salt

⅛ teaspoon freshly ground black pepper

½ cup shredded cheddar cheese

4 tablespoons sour cream, divided

2 scallions, white parts only, thinly sliced

Per Serving (2 pieces, topped): Calories: 159; Total fat: 13g; Total carbs: 5g; Fiber: 1g; Net carbs: 4g; Protein: 8g; Macronutrients: Fat: 70%; Protein: 19%; Carbs: 11%

1. Preheat the oven to 400°F. Rub each zucchini with 1 teaspoon of oil.
2. Lay the zucchini on a baking sheet and bake for 10 minutes. Remove from the oven and allow to cool completely.
3. Reduce the oven heat to 350°F and line a baking sheet with parchment paper. Line a plate with paper towels.
4. Lay the bacon slices in a single layer on the prepared baking sheet and bake for 12 minutes. Remove from the oven and drain the bacon on the prepared plate. Increase the oven heat to 450°F.
5. When the bacon is cool enough to handle, crumble it into pieces.
6. Cut the cooled zucchini in half horizontally, and then again lengthwise. Scoop out the inside of each zucchini half, leaving about ¼ inch of flesh.
7. Season the insides of each zucchini "skin" with salt and pepper. Place the zucchini skin-side down in a baking dish and bake for 7 minutes. Flip and bake for another 7 minutes.

8. Remove from the oven and turn the heat to broil.

9. Cover each zucchini skin with equal amounts of cheese and bacon crumbles. Broil for 60 to 90 seconds, or until the cheese is bubbly.

10. Top each skin with ½ tablespoon of sour cream and equal amounts of scallion.

11. Serve immediately.

SUBSTITUTION TIP: These zucchini skins are a great vessel for adding more low-carb greens. Take ⅓ cup of steamed broccoli or cauliflower—or a mix—and add them equally to each zucchini skin. Top with the cheese and bacon and broil until bubbly.

Margarita Pizza Chips

SERVES 8 | PREP TIME: 10 MINUTES | COOK TIME: 10 MINUTES

Is it a chip? Is it pizza? Oh, hooray—it's both! Pizza and chips were on the menu at every after-school playdate, birthday party, and sleepover I had growing up. This recipe removes all the starch by replacing pizza dough with savory salami to give you a zesty keto appetizer. Draining off the excess oil after cooking provides a tasty, crunchy bite.

16 slices deli salami
2 medium tomatoes, cut
   into ¼-inch-thick slices
Pinch salt
Pinch pepper
8 ounces fresh mozzarella,
   cut into 16 pieces
16 fresh basil leaves

Per Serving: Calories: 155; Total fat: 12g; Total carbs: 1g; Fiber: <1g; Net carbs: 1g; Protein: 9g; Macronutrients: Fat: 72%; Protein: 25%; Carbs: 3%

1. Preheat the oven to 375°F. Line a rimmed baking sheet with parchment paper. Line a plate with paper towels.
2. Lay the salami on the parchment paper and bake for 9 minutes, until the salami browns on the edges and begins to shrink.
3. While the salami bakes, season the tomatoes with salt and pepper and set aside.
4. Once the salami is done, transfer it to the prepared plate to drain excess oil for a couple of minutes. Turn the oven to broil.
5. Place the crisp salami on the prepared baking sheet. Top each slice with a slice of tomato, a basil leaf, and a mozzarella slice.
6. Return the baking sheet to the oven and broil for 60 to 90 seconds, until the cheese begins to bubble.
7. Allow the bites to cool for 2 to 3 minutes, then transfer to a dish and serve.

> **PREPARATION TIP:** Once you remove the bites from the broiler, if they're a little oily, simply move them to a paper towel for a few minutes.

Mozzarella Sticks

SERVES 4 | PREP TIME: 10 MINUTES, PLUS 2 HOURS TO CHILL | COOK TIME: 10 MINUTES

Mozzarella cheese is salty, creamy, and perfectly ooey-gooey. Although a baked version of these sticks will not yield the same crisp as frying does, the flavor remains intact, and cleanup is a cinch. Every mozzarella stick deserves a delicious dunk, so consider serving these with ranch dressing or Marinara Sauce (page 154).

6 sticks whole-milk mozzarella string cheese, halved
1 tablespoon coconut flour
1 tablespoon almond flour
¼ cup crushed pork rinds
¼ cup parmesan cheese
1 teaspoon dried Italian seasoning
1 large egg
Olive oil cooking spray

Per Serving (3 pieces): Calories: 212; Total fat: 16g; Total carbs: 3g; Fiber: 1g; Net carbs: 2g; Protein: 16g; Macronutrients: Fat: 65%; Protein: 31%; Carbs: 4%

1. Line a baking sheet with parchment paper. Lay the mozzarella pieces on the baking sheet in a single layer and freeze for 1 hour.

2. In a medium bowl, whisk together the coconut flour, almond flour, pork rinds, parmesan, and Italian seasoning. Pour the mixture out into a shallow dish.

3. In another shallow dish, beat the egg.

4. Dip each frozen mozzarella piece in the egg and then roll it in the flour mixture to coat completely. Return the pieces to the baking sheet and freeze again for 1 hour.

5. Preheat the oven to 450°F. Spray each piece of coated mozzarella with cooking spray. Bake for 5 minutes, flip, and lightly spray with cooking spray again. Bake for another 5 minutes.

6. Allow the mozzarella to cool slightly before eating. Refrigerate leftovers for up to 3 days and reheat on the stovetop in a dry nonstick frying pan until heated through.

MAKE AHEAD: Follow steps 1 to 4. After the hour of freezing, move them into an airtight container, separating layers with parchment paper. Freeze for up to 1 month.

Jalapeño Poppers

SERVES 4 | PREP TIME: 15 MINUTES | COOK TIME: 20 MINUTES

Spicy, cheesy, and crunchy, jalapeño poppers hit the spot. The poppers you find at restaurants are deep fried, but these are wrapped in bacon and baked. The mess is nonexistent, and the crunch and flavor are spot-on. These are great for making in bulk for feeding a crowd.

4 jalapeño peppers, halved and seeded

4 ounces softened full-fat cream cheese

⅓ cup shredded cheddar cheese

4 slices bacon, halved horizontally

2 tablespoons sour cream

Per Serving (2 pepper halves): Calories: 189; Total fat: 17g; Total carbs: 3g; Fiber: <1g; Net carbs: 3g; Protein: 7g; Macronutrients: Fat: 78%; Protein: 15%; Carbs: 7%

1. Preheat the oven to 375°F. Line a baking sheet with parchment paper.
2. Place the pepper halves on the prepared baking sheet.
3. In a small bowl, mix together the cream cheese and cheddar until well combined.
4. Spoon the cheese mixture evenly into each pepper half.
5. Wrap each jalapeño half with a piece of bacon and secure with a toothpick.
6. Bake for 15 to 20 minutes or until the bacon is crisp.
7. Top each pepper half with sour cream. Serve immediately. Jalapeño poppers can be refrigerated for up to 3 days, but without the sour cream on top as it does not reheat well.

PREPARATION TIP: Protect your eyes, wear gloves when handling the peppers, and wash your hands thoroughly. Don't touch your eyes after touching a jalapeño pepper with bare hands.

Deviled Eggs

SERVES 4 | PREP TIME: 20 MINUTES | COOK TIME: 10 MINUTES

A great thing about deviled eggs is being able to make a big batch and play with the flavor, adding different ingredients and toppings. This recipe with avocado oil mayonnaise and butter provides a rich, creamy base to build on. These are delicious on their own, but experiment with added spice from hot sauce or sriracha, or combine flavors like bacon, ranch, and cheddar. These deviled eggs are your creamy blank canvas.

6 large eggs
1 tablespoon plus
⅛ teaspoon sea
salt, divided
3 tablespoons avocado
oil mayonnaise
1 tablespoon butter, at
room temperature
2 teaspoons Dijon mustard
¼ teaspoon paprika

Per Serving (3 deviled eggs): Calories: 146; Total fat: 13g; Total carbs: 1g; Fiber: <1g; Net carbs: 1g; Protein: 6g; Macronutrients: Fat: 79%; Protein: 19%; Carbs: 2%

1. In a medium saucepan over high heat, completely submerge the eggs in cold water.
2. Add 1 tablespoon of salt and bring the water to a boil.
3. As soon as it begins to boil, turn the heat off but do not remove the pan from the stove. Cover it and set a timer for 13 minutes. (If the eggs are just-from-the-farm fresh, set it for 11 minutes.)
4. Prepare an ice bath with 2 to 3 cups of cold water and 10 ice cubes. When the timer goes off, carefully remove the eggs with a slotted spoon and transfer straight to the ice bath, submerging them completely. Let them cool for 4 to 5 minutes.
5. Gently crack the eggshells on a hard surface and then slide the shells off. Rinse to get rid of all shell remnants.
6. Slice each egg in half and scoop the yolk out into a medium bowl. Set the whites aside on a plate.
7. Add the mayonnaise, butter, Dijon, and remaining ⅛ teaspoon of salt to the yolks. Mash with a fork and stir until well combined and creamy.
8. Spoon the yolk mixture evenly into each egg white. Sprinkle with the paprika and serve immediately or refrigerate for up to 2 days.

BLT Sandwich

SERVES 2 | PREP TIME: 10 MINUTES | COOK TIME: 20 MINUTES

Crunchy, salty bacon smashed between fresh tomato, crispy lettuce, tangy mayonnaise, and chewy bread, a BLT is my favorite sandwich. The key to a perfect BLT is the bacon—lots of it. Avocado oil mayonnaise and avocado slices add another layer of richness to form a creamy, savory, crunchy sandwich.

12 slices bacon

2 batches 90-Second Bread (page 158)

2 tablespoons avocado oil mayonnaise, divided

4 iceberg lettuce leaves

4 slices tomato

1 small Haas avocado, sliced

Per Serving (1 sandwich): Calories: 750; Total fat: 67g; Total carbs: 14g; Fiber: 8g; Net carbs: 6g; Protein: 29g; Macronutrients: Fat: 77%; Protein: 16%; Carbs: 7%

1. Preheat the oven to 350°F. Line a rimmed baking sheet with parchment paper. Line a plate with paper towels.

2. Lay the bacon slices in a single layer on the parchment paper. Make sure the slices do not overlap. Bake for 20 to 23 minutes, or until as crispy as you like.

3. Transfer the bacon to the prepared plate.

4. Make the 90-Second Bread. When each piece is cool enough to handle, slice in half and toast.

5. Slather each slice of toast with ½ tablespoon of mayonnaise. Layer 2 pieces of toast with lettuce leaves, tomato slices, avocado, and bacon, and top with the remaining slices of toast. Enjoy!

Grilled Cheese Sandwich

SERVES 1 | PREP TIME: 15 MINUTES | COOK TIME: 10 MINUTES

There are restaurants devoted just to this one sandwich—and for a good reason. Grilled cheese is nothing short of ubiquitous because of how many flavor combinations there are. Some of my favorites include pepper Jack with tomato and Brie with ham and mustard. You can use just about any cheese, though I find that hard cheeses don't melt as well. Serve with Creamy Tomato Soup (page 45) to feel a big hug from the inside.

1 batch 90-Second Bread (page 158)
Cooking spray
1 tablespoon avocado oil mayonnaise, divided
2 ounces American cheese

Per Serving (1 sandwich): Calories: 608; Total fat: 57g; Total carbs: 8g; Fiber: 2g; Net carbs: 6g; Protein: 21g; Macronutrients: Fat: 81%; Protein: 14%; Carbs: 5%

1. Make the 90-Second Bread. When each piece is cool enough to handle, slice in half and toast.
2. Spray a small frying pan with cooking spray and place it on medium-low heat. Slather ½ tablespoon of mayonnaise on each piece of toast.
3. Place 1 slice of bread, mayo-side down, in the pan. Top it with the cheese, and put the other slice of bread on top, mayo-side up.
4. When the cheese begins to melt, flip the sandwich and cook until golden, about 3 minutes more.
5. Slice in half and serve immediately.

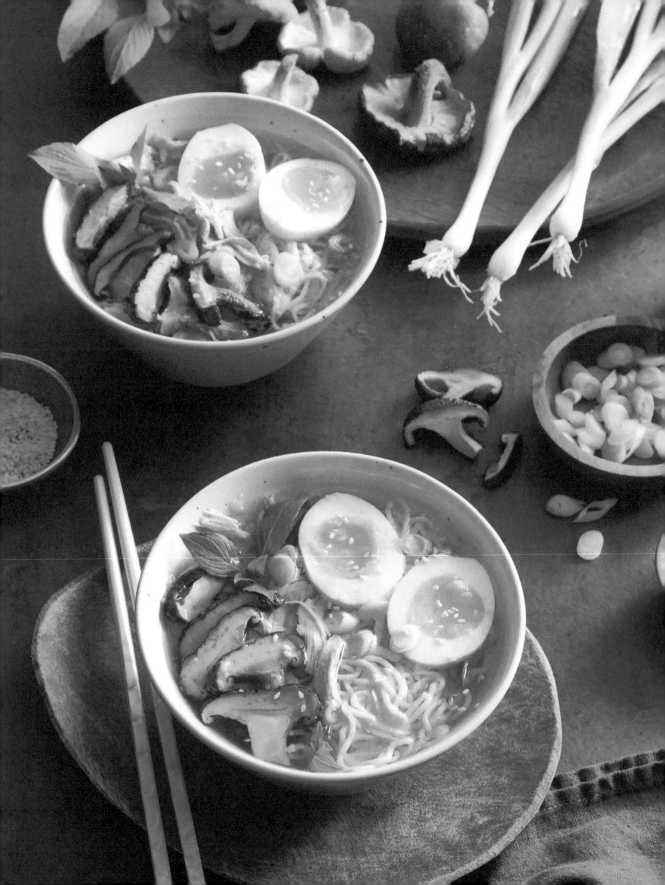

Chicken Ramen Soup

SERVES 4 | PREP TIME: 25 MINUTES | COOK TIME: 30 MINUTES

Traditional Japanese ramen includes broth, meat, vegetables, and non-keto-friendly noodles. This recipe packs the same savory punch as the thrifty soup you may have had during college or growing up but replaces the starchy dried noodles with shirataki noodles. If you cannot find coconut aminos, use low-sodium soy sauce.

2 packages
  shirataki noodles
4 ounces
  shiitake mushrooms
1 teaspoon avocado oil
½ teaspoon sea salt
4 chicken bouillon cubes
4 cups water
1 tablespoon olive oil
2 garlic cloves, minced
¼ teaspoon ground ginger
3½ tablespoons
  shredded carrots
2½ tablespoons
  coconut aminos
2 cups shredded
  rotisserie chicken
4 soft boiled eggs, halved
1 scallion, white part only,
  diced (optional)
Hot sauce (optional)

Per Serving (1 cup): Calories: 275; Total fat: 12g; Total carbs: 13g; Fiber: 7g; Net carbs: 6g; Protein: 21g; Macronutrients: Fat: 43%; Protein: 40%; Carbs: 17%

1. Preheat the oven to 400°F. Line a baking sheet with paper towels. Line a baking sheet with parchment paper.

2. Rinse and drain the noodles thoroughly. Place them on the prepared baking sheet and cover with more paper towels. Gently press to soak up the water. Discard the top layer of paper towels and let the noodles air-dry for 20 minutes.

3. Place the mushrooms (stems and caps) on the parchment paper–lined baking sheet and drizzle evenly with the avocado oil. Sprinkle with the salt. Bake for 20 minutes. Set aside.

4. In a medium saucepan over medium-high heat, warm the bouillon cubes and water together until the bouillon dissolves. Turn off the heat.

5. Pour the olive oil into a large saucepan over medium heat. Add the garlic, ginger, and carrots, stirring frequently so the garlic does not burn. Cook until fragrant, 1 to 2 minutes.

6. Add the noodles and stir-fry for another 2 to 3 minutes.

CONTINUED ▶

7. Add the bouillon, coconut aminos, and chicken. Bring the mixture to a boil and then reduce the heat to low and simmer for 5 minutes.

8. Divide the soup equally into four bowls. Top each bowl of ramen with a halved egg, equal portions of mushrooms, and equal portions of scallions (if using). Drizzle with hot sauce (if using).

> **SUBSTITUTION TIP:** Swap the chicken bouillon for beef bouillon and trade the chicken for 1 pound cooked, sliced flank steak. Or go vegetarian by using vegetable bouillon and using 2 cups of bok choy instead of chicken.

Creamy Tomato Soup

SERVES 3 | PREP TIME: 5 MINUTES | COOK TIME: 15 MINUTES

I remember a soup commercial of a little snowman playing outside. When it was time to eat, he sat at the table while his mother served him a warm bowl of tomato soup. The ice and snow quickly melted to reveal a happy little boy, enjoying his soup. Creamy tomato soup does exactly that: it melts away the cold and leaves us warm, happy, and comforted.

1 (14.5-ounce) can diced unsalted tomatoes
1 cup chicken bone broth
½ teaspoon salt
¼ teaspoon dried thyme
¼ teaspoon garlic powder
Pinch ground nutmeg
¼ cup heavy cream
Freshly ground black pepper (optional)

Per Serving: Calories: 119; Total fat: 8g; Total carbs: 8g; Fiber: 2g; Net carbs: 6g; Protein: 5g; Macronutrients: Fat: 55%; Protein: 18%; Carbs: 27%

1. In a medium saucepan over medium-high heat, combine the tomatoes, broth, salt, thyme, garlic powder, and nutmeg. Bring to a boil and then reduce the heat to low and simmer for 5 minutes.
2. Either with an immersion blender or in a regular blender, puree the soup.
3. Pour the soup back into the saucepan and turn the heat to medium low.
4. Slowly whisk in the cream and continue whisking until well combined. Simmer for 5 more minutes.
5. Portion into bowls and serve. Season with pepper (if using). Refrigerate for up to 2 days or freeze for up to 1 month.

SUBSTITUTION TIP: If you do not have bone broth, regular chicken broth works, too. If you're not using low-sodium broth, remove the salt this recipe calls for and simply add salt to taste before serving.

Hearty Cauliflower Soup

MAKES 4 CUPS | PREP TIME: 10 MINUTES | COOK TIME: 50 MINUTES

Creamy, hearty soups fill the belly and warm the heart. By using low-carb cauliflower, buttery mascarpone cheese, and heavy cream, this soup is everything a keto comfort soup should be. Mascarpone is best for its richness, but you can also use full-fat cream cheese. No bone broth? Simply use low-sodium chicken broth. You really can't go wrong with this hearty soup.

4 cups cauliflower florets
¼ cup melted butter
¼ teaspoon sea salt
1 tablespoon olive oil
1 garlic clove, minced
¼ cup diced white onion
Pinch ground nutmeg
⅛ teaspoon thyme
2 cups chicken bone broth
2 tablespoons mascarpone, at room temperature, divided
¼ cup heavy cream
Sea salt
Freshly ground black pepper

Per Serving (1 cup): Calories: 271; Total fat: 24g; Total carbs: 7g; Fiber: 2g; Net carbs: 5g; Protein: 8g; Macronutrients: Fat: 79%; Protein: 11%; Carbs: 10%

1. Preheat the oven to 375°F. Line a baking sheet with parchment paper.
2. In a large bowl, toss the cauliflower, butter, and salt together until well combined.
3. Pour the cauliflower onto the prepared baking sheet in a single layer. Bake for 30 minutes, until the cauliflower is fork-tender and begins to brown.
4. In a large saucepan over medium-low heat, heat the olive oil. Add the garlic, stirring frequently, and cook for about 45 seconds. Stir in the onion, sprinkle in the nutmeg and thyme, and cook for another 5 to 7 minutes, until the onions are translucent.
5. Transfer the roasted cauliflower to the saucepan. Stir together.
6. Add the chicken broth and bring the soup to a boil. Reduce the heat to medium low and simmer for 15 to 20 minutes, until all the vegetables are soft.

7. Stir in the mascarpone ½ tablespoon at a time until melted.

8. Slowly add the heavy cream, stirring constantly, until it is thoroughly incorporated. Season with salt and pepper.

9. Transfer three-fourths of the soup to a blender and blend until smooth.

10. Pour the blended soup back into the saucepan and stir to combine. This method uses the soup itself as a thickener.

11. Portion into bowls and serve. Refrigerate leftovers for up to 4 days or freeze for up to 3 months.

> **SUBSTITUTION TIP:** Create a version of loaded baked potato soup by topping each bowl with a cooked, crumbled piece of bacon, 1 tablespoon of shredded cheddar cheese, ½ tablespoon of sour cream, and 1 teaspoon of chopped scallion.

Broccoli Cheese Soup

MAKES 4 CUPS | PREP TIME: 5 MINUTES | COOK TIME: 40 MINUTES

What I look for in a good broccoli cheese soup is chunks of fresh broccoli, a strong cheese taste, and a hearty texture. That is exactly what this recipe delivers: a thick, creamy broccoli-forward bowl of soup that is stick-to-your-ribs filling.

4 tablespoons
   unsalted butter
1 garlic clove, minced
¼ cup diced white onion
4 cups broccoli florets
3 cups chicken bone broth
2 tablespoons full-fat
   cream cheese, at
   room temperature
¼ cup heavy cream
1¼ cups shredded cheddar
   cheese, divided

Per Serving (1 cup): Calories: 384; Total fat: 31g; Total carbs: 8g; Fiber: 2g; Net carbs: 6g; Protein: 19g; Macronutrients: Fat: 72%; Protein: 20%; Carbs: 8%

1. In a large saucepan over medium heat, melt the butter, swirling it to coat the pan completely.
2. Stir in the garlic and onion and cook until translucent, about 3 minutes.
3. Stir in the broccoli and cook for another 2 minutes, stirring frequently.
4. Pour in the broth and turn the heat to high. Once it begins to boil, drop the heat to medium low and simmer for 25 to 30 minutes, until the broccoli is tender. Drop the heat to low.
5. Cut the cream cheese into chunks and slowly stir it into the soup. Stir well to allow the cheese to melt and become completely incorporated. Slowly add the cream, whisking so the mixture does not separate.
6. Next, stir in the cheddar ¼ cup at a time, allowing it to melt completely before adding more. This ensures that all the cheese fully incorporates to provide a creamy texture.

7. Use a ladle to transfer half of the soup to a blender. Blend to puree. Pour the pureed soup back into the saucepan and stir well to incorporate. This method thickens the soup while also leaving chunks of fresh broccoli.

8. Divide the soup into bowls, or refrigerate for up to 3 days.

MAKE AHEAD: This recipe is an easy one to set and forget in your slow cooker. Follow steps 1 to 3; then add the broth, cover, and cook on high for 3 hours or low for 6 hours. If you want to use frozen broccoli, reduce the bone broth to 2¼ cups. Low-sodium chicken broth also works here.

Chicken Noodle Soup

SERVES 4 | PREP TIME: 20 MINUTES | COOK TIME: 15 MINUTES

This soul-satisfying soup is loaded with nutrients from fresh vegetables and bone broth, and it's simple to throw together. Chicken noodle soup can also be a great way to use up any leftover veggies you have on hand. Just sauté them with the garlic, onion, and celery for an even more filling dish.

2 tablespoons olive oil
2 baby carrots, diced
1 garlic clove, minced
¼ cup diced white onion
2 celery stalks, diced
4 cups chicken bone broth
2 cups shredded
  rotisserie chicken
½ teaspoon dried thyme
½ teaspoon dried oregano
2 cups Zoodles (page 166)
Sea salt
Freshly ground
  black pepper

Per Serving (1¼ cups):
Calories: 266; Total fat: 11g;
Total carbs: 8g; Fiber: 2g;
Net carbs: 6g; Protein: 26g;
Macronutrients: Fat: 41%;
Protein: 49%; Carbs: 10%

1. In a large saucepan over medium heat, heat the olive oil. Add the carrots and cook for 2 minutes.
2. Stir in the garlic, onion, and celery and cook until softened, about 5 minutes.
3. Stir in the broth, chicken, thyme, and oregano until well combined. Add the zoodles and stir again.
4. Bring the soup to a boil; then reduce the heat to low and simmer for about 7 minutes or until the zoodles are cooked but still have a little crunch. Season with salt and pepper to taste.
5. Divide the soup into bowls and serve immediately. Refrigerate leftovers for up to 4 days or freeze for up to 3 months.

MAKE AHEAD: Make your own shredded chicken in a slow cooker by combining 3 pounds of boneless chicken breast or thighs, 4 tablespoons of unsalted butter (chopped), and 1½ to 2 cups of chicken bone broth or low-sodium chicken stock. Cover and cook on high for 3 hours or low for 6 hours. Shred the chicken and place in an airtight container. Pour some of the cooking juices over top and refrigerate for up to 5 days. This doesn't freeze well.

Italian Garden Salad

SERVES 4 | PREP TIME: 15 MINUTES

A salad may not be on your comfort foods list—but your opinion might change after trying this one. The creamy Italian-style dressing is the perfect tangy topper to an array of crunchy low-carb veggies. Olives and parmesan cheese provide the healthy fats to keep you feeling full. Serve this with a hearty soup or make a batch of breadsticks from Cauliflower Dough (page 161) for a truly satisfying meal.

¼ cup olive oil

2 tablespoons white vinegar

2 tablespoons avocado oil mayonnaise

1 teaspoon dried Italian seasoning

½ teaspoon garlic powder

¼ teaspoon sea salt

⅛ teaspoon freshly ground black pepper

1 batch 90-Second Bread (page 158; see Note)

2 cups chopped romaine lettuce

4 tablespoons sliced black olives

2 small Roma tomatoes, sliced

¼ cup thinly sliced red onion

¼ cup chopped green bell pepper

⅓ cup parmesan cheese

Per Serving (1 cup): Calories: 309; Total fat: 30g; Total carbs: 6g; Fiber: 2g; Net carbs: 4g; Protein: 6g; Macronutrients: Fat: 85%; Protein: 8%; Carbs: 7%

1. In a medium bowl, whisk together the oil, vinegar, mayonnaise, Italian seasoning, garlic powder, salt, and pepper until well combined. Set aside.
2. Make the 90-Second Bread. When each piece is cool enough to handle, slice in half and toast on a medium-high setting. Cut the toast into small cubes.
3. In a large bowl, toss together the lettuce, olives, tomatoes, onion, and bell pepper. Add the croutons and toss again.
4. Pour in the dressing and toss until the vegetables are completely coated. Stir in the parmesan cheese.
5. Divide the salad into bowls and serve immediately.

NOTE: Make the 90-Second Bread with 1 tablespoon olive oil in lieu of the butter and the addition of ⅛ teaspoon garlic powder and ⅛ teaspoon dried oregano to the batter.

FEEDING THE FAMILY: Top each serving with 4 ounces of cooked chicken, steak, shrimp, or salmon for a complete, filling meal.

Cobb Salad

Cobb salads are simple to make and can be assembled in minutes, leaving you full, happy, and ready to get on with your day. I love the acidity of red wine vinegar and the tang it adds. It's an added bonus that red wine vinegar is a zero-carb flavor option. Feel free to trade the chicken for your favorite protein and swap the blue cheese crumbles for your favorite shredded cheese.

1½ tablespoons olive oil

2 teaspoons red wine vinegar

2 cups chopped romaine lettuce

½ cup chopped cucumber

1 small Roma tomato, chopped

½ cup cooked, shredded chicken

1 hardboiled egg, chopped

2 slices bacon, cooked and crumbled

½ small Haas avocado, sliced

2 tablespoons crumbled blue cheese

Sea salt

Freshly ground black pepper

1. In a small bowl, whisk together the oil and vinegar. Set aside.
2. Arrange the lettuce on a large dish or in a deep bowl. Spread the cucumber along the right side of the lettuce. Lay the tomato in a single layer next to the cucumber.
3. Place the chicken in the middle of the dish, then arrange lines of egg, bacon, avocado, and blue cheese crumbles. This salad is looking beautiful.
4. Whisk the olive oil and vinegar one more time and then drizzle on top of the salad.
5. Season with salt and pepper and serve.

Per Serving (1 salad): Calories: 660; Total fat: 47g; Total carbs: 16g; Fiber: 8g; Net carbs: 8g; Protein: 47g; Macronutrients: Fat: 63%; Protein: 29%; Carbs: 8%

Ground Beef Tacos

SERVES 4 | PREP TIME: 10 MINUTES | COOK TIME: 10 MINUTES

Tacos are my desert island food. These replace the corn tortilla with a cheesy taco shell. You can omit the cheese and use lettuce leaves as taco shells, or serve the ground taco meat over chopped lettuce.

1 cup shredded cheddar cheese, divided
1 pound 80/20 ground beef
1 teaspoon sea salt
½ teaspoon ground cumin
½ teaspoon ground coriander
½ teaspoon paprika
¼ teaspoon garlic powder
¼ teaspoon dried oregano
⅛ teaspoon chili powder
⅛ teaspoon ground black pepper
½ cup water

OPTIONAL TOPPINGS
Shredded lettuce
Sour cream
Shredded cheese
Avocado

Per Serving (2 tacos): Calories: 402; Total fat: 28g; Total carbs: 2g; Fiber: <1g; Net carbs: 2g; Protein: 36g; Macronutrients: Fat: 61%; Protein: 37%; Carbs: 2%

1. Preheat the oven to 375°F. Line a baking sheet with parchment paper.
2. Place ¼ cup of cheese at a time onto the baking sheet and form into circles. Bake for 5 to 7 minutes, checking the cheese frequently to prevent burning.
3. While the cheese bakes, create a taco mold by positioning two equal-size glasses across from one another with a wooden spoon resting on top.
4. Remove the cheese circles from the oven and let them cool for 1 minute. With a spatula, transfer each circle to hang over the wooden spoon.
5. While the cheese shells are hardening, place a large saucepan over medium heat. Cook the ground beef until browned, about 5 minutes.
6. Remove from the heat, drain the fat, and put the pan back on the heat. Add the salt, cumin, coriander, paprika, garlic powder, oregano, chili powder, and black pepper and stir well to combine. Pour in the water and stir again.

CONTINUED

7. Bring to a boil; then reduce the heat to medium-low and simmer until the water is gone, 5 to 6 more minutes.

8. To serve, fill each taco shell with one-fourth of the ground beef and top with your desired toppings.

> **SUBSTITUTION TIP:** To make nachos, cut the hardened cheese into chips.

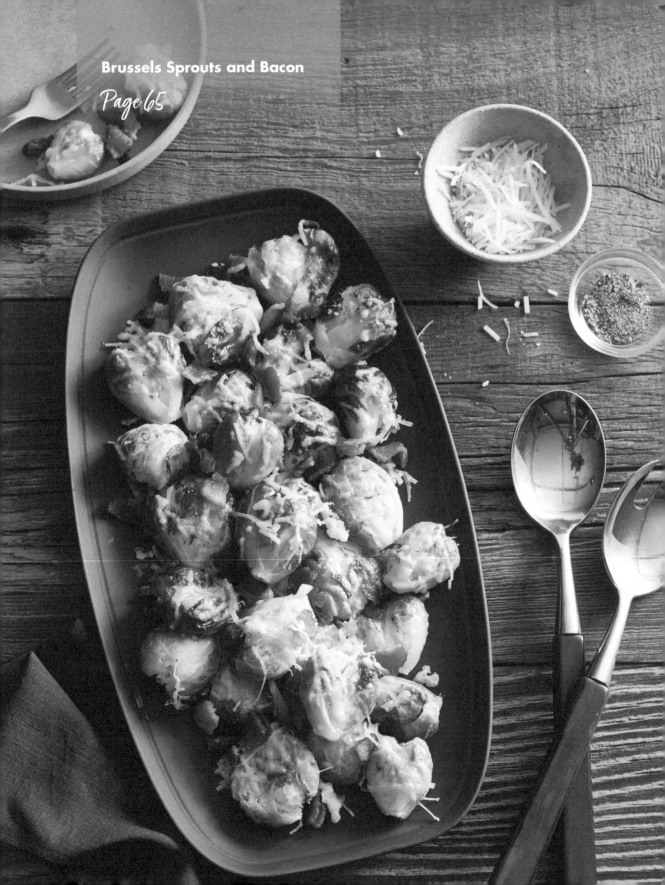

Brussels Sprouts and Bacon

Page 65

Chapter 4

VEGETABLES

Buttery Caulimash

SERVES 4 | PREP TIME: 5 MINUTES | COOK TIME: 20 MINUTES

If creamy mashed potatoes are the carb-loaded mother of all comfort food vegetable dishes, buttery caulimash is her keto-friendly daughter. Warm, buttery, savory, and filling, this recipe pairs well with any protein. The mascarpone cheese adds to the dish's creaminess but doesn't taste like cheese. If you can't find mascarpone, cream cheese or sour cream both work well.

4 cups cauliflower florets
4 tablespoons butter, at room temperature
2 tablespoons mascarpone cheese, at room temperature
½ teaspoon sea salt
⅛ teaspoon freshly ground black pepper

Per Serving (⅔ cup): Calories: 182; Total fat: 18g; Total carbs: 4g; Fiber: 2g; Net carbs: 2g; Protein: 3g; Macronutrients: Fat: 87%; Protein: 6%; Carbs: 7%

1. Fill a large frying pan over medium-high heat with ¼ inch of water. Bring the water to a boil and then add the cauliflower florets.
2. Cover and steam the cauliflower for 15 minutes until soft. Transfer the cauliflower to a blender.
3. Add the butter, cheese, salt, and pepper and blend until pureed. Serve.
4. Refrigerate leftovers for up to 3 days.

Cauliflower Mac and Cheese

SERVES 4 | PREP TIME: 10 MINUTES | COOK TIME: 35 MINUTES

Eaten as a side or main course, dressed up with lobster or right out of a box, just about everyone loves a hearty helping of macaroni and cheese. With its ooey-gooey, fat-filled, and low-carb cheese, regular mac and cheese is halfway to being a keto-friendly food. Replacing the pasta with cauliflower takes care of the rest.

1¼ cups roughly chopped cauliflower florets

4 ounces mascarpone cheese, at room temperature

½ cup heavy cream

½ cup full-fat sour cream

½ cup shredded cheddar cheese, divided

1 teaspoon sea salt

¼ teaspoon garlic powder

⅛ teaspoon paprika

Per Serving (⅓ cup): Calories: 344; Total fat: 34g; Total carbs: 5g; Fiber: 1g; Net carbs: 4g; Protein: 8g; Macronutrients: Fat: 87%; Protein: 9%; Carbs: 4%

1. Preheat the oven to 350°F.
2. Fill a large frying pan over medium-high heat with ¼ inch of water. Bring the water to a boil and then add the cauliflower florets. Cover and steam for 10 minutes, until the cauliflower is fork-tender but not completely soft.
3. In a large bowl, combine the mascarpone, cream, sour cream, ¼ cup of cheddar, salt, garlic powder, and paprika.
4. Stir in the cauliflower to completely coat it. Transfer to a small baking dish and top with the remaining ¼ cup of cheddar.
5. Bake for 22 to 25 minutes, until the cheese is lightly browned. Serve, or refrigerate for up to 3 days.

SUBSTITUTION TIP: Swap the mascarpone for cream cheese and add 2 tablespoons of ranch dressing in step 2. Once the dish is baked, top it with cooked, crumbled bacon and chopped scallions.

Collard Greens with Ham

SERVES 4 | PREP TIME: 10 MINUTES | COOK TIME: 1 HOUR 25 MINUTES

The first time I ate collard greens was when I moved close to a barbecue restaurant. I found them quite unpleasant. During a girls' weekend in Savannah, I tried them again, and this time they were cooked down and flavored with pork. Now I love them. This recipe is lightly kissed with smoke from the ham and spice from the hot sauce.

1 tablespoon coconut oil
¼ cup diced white onion
1¼ cups cubed ham
2 cups collard greens, stemmed and roughly chopped
½ teaspoon garlic powder
¼ teaspoon freshly ground black pepper
2 cups chicken broth
¼ cup apple cider vinegar
½ teaspoon hot sauce (optional)

Per Serving (¾ cup): Calories: 121; Total fat: 6g; Total carbs: 5g; Fiber: 1g; Net carbs: 4g; Protein: 10g; Macronutrients: Fat: 46%; Protein: 34%; Carbs: 20%

1. Heat the oil in a large soup pot over medium heat. Add the onion and cook for 3 to 5 minutes, until translucent.
2. Stir in the ham and cook until it begins to brown, stirring frequently so the onion does not burn.
3. Drop the greens in, one handful at a time, stirring after each handful and allowing the leaves to begin to wilt before adding another handful. This will take 7 to 10 minutes.
4. Add the garlic powder, pepper, broth, and vinegar. Stir to combine. Bring to a boil and then drop the heat to low.
5. Cover and simmer for 1 to 1½ hours, checking every 20 minutes, until the greens are tender. Add some water, ½ cup at a time, if necessary.
6. Add the hot sauce (if using) and stir well. Serve or refrigerate for up to 4 days.

SUBSTITUTION TIP: Replace the ham with 1 pound of chopped bacon. Fry the bacon pieces first. When cooked, but not yet crisp, remove with a slotted spoon and drain on a paper towel–lined plate. Reserve the grease and use it in place of the coconut oil. Once the onions are translucent, return the bacon to the pan and follow the remaining steps.

Jicama Fries

SERVES 4 | PREP TIME: 30 MINUTES | COOK TIME: 35 MINUTES

French fries are the ultimate side dish—or even entrée depending on whom you're talking to (hello, me). Carb-heavy potatoes are far from keto-friendly, but another root vegetable can provide that crunchy bite: jicama. Jicama is low in carbohydrates with the snap of a crisp potato fry. Soaking the jicama in boiling water first helps keep the crunch.

2 cups fresh jicama, cut into fries
4 cups water
2 teaspoons sea salt, divided
1 teaspoon garlic powder
1 teaspoon onion powder
2 tablespoons avocado oil
1 teaspoon dried parsley

Per Serving (½ cup): Calories: 72; Total fat: 7g; Total carbs: 3g; Fiber: 1g; Net carbs: 2g; Protein: <1g; Macronutrients: Fat: 84%; Protein: 1%; Carbs: 15%

1. Preheat the oven to 400°F. Line a baking sheet with paper towels.
2. Put the jicama in a large bowl. Bring the water to a boil and then pour it directly over the jicama. Let sit for 20 minutes.
3. Drain the jicama and transfer to the prepared baking sheet (toss the paper towels). Cover with more paper towels to absorb as much water as possible (this helps with crispiness).
4. Return the jicama to the bowl and toss with 1 teaspoon of salt, the garlic powder, the onion powder, and the oil.
5. Spread the jicama fries in an even layer on the baking sheet.
6. Bake for 15 minutes, flip, and cook for another 15 to 20 minutes or until crisp.
7. Toss the cooked jicama fries with remaining 1 teaspoon salt and dried parsley.
8. Serve immediately or store in a single layer in an airtight container for up to 2 days. Reheat under a broiler for 1 to 2 minutes.

PREPARATION TIP: Many stores carry raw, sliced jicama in the produce section, so you can speed up the prep.

Zucchini Fries

SERVES 4 | PREP TIME: 20 MINUTES | COOK TIME: 25 MINUTES

Think of zucchini fries as keto-friendly steak fries. Almond flour and parmesan develop a crispy exterior to these zucchini fries. Eating them is just like biting into a deep-fried steak fry but without all the carbs. To make these dairy-free, replace the parmesan with crushed pork rinds. The cooking time remains the same, and they will be just as crunchy.

2 large zucchini, halved lengthwise and cut into ½-inch strips
1 teaspoon sea salt
1 large egg
1 tablespoon coconut flour
⅓ cup almond flour
¼ cup finely grated parmesan cheese
¼ teaspoon garlic powder
¼ teaspoon dried rosemary

Per Serving (½ zucchini): Calories: 134; Total fat: 9g; Total carbs: 9g; Fiber: 3g; Net carbs: 6g; Protein: 8g; Macronutrients: Fat: 54%; Protein: 20%; Carbs: 26%

1. Preheat the oven to 425°F. Line a baking sheet with paper towels. Line a second baking sheet with parchment paper.

2. Lay the zucchini strips on the paper towels. Sprinkle with the sea salt and let sit for 15 minutes.

3. In a small bowl, beat the egg. Put the coconut flour in another small bowl. In a large, shallow dish, combine the almond flour, parmesan, garlic powder, and rosemary.

4. Pat the zucchini slices dry with paper towels. Dredge them first in coconut flour, then egg, and then almond flour. Lay them one by one on the parchment paper. Do not overlap!

5. Bake for 15 minutes. Flip and bake for another 10 minutes. Let cool slightly before devouring.

Scalloped Zucchini

SERVES 6 | PREP TIME: 15 MINUTES | COOK TIME: 55 MINUTES

Cauliflower is often praised as the perfect low-carb swap for potatoes, but when it comes to making a rich and cheesy scalloped dish, zucchini reigns supreme. Unlike scalloped potatoes that are somewhat complicated and take a long time to cook, this dish is ready in a little over an hour. The Brie cheese adds an extra layer of buttery, cheesy flavor.

3 medium zucchini, cut into thin disks

½ teaspoon sea salt

2 tablespoons butter

2 garlic cloves, minced

2 ounces full-fat cream cheese, at room temperature

⅔ cup shredded mozzarella, divided

4 ounces Brie cheese, sliced

¼ cup heavy cream

½ teaspoon dried Italian seasoning

¼ teaspoon freshly ground black pepper

Pinch nutmeg

Cooking spray

Per Serving (⅓ cup): Calories: 222; Total fat: 19g; Total carbs: 5g; Fiber: 1g; Net carbs: 4g; Protein: 9g; Macronutrients: Fat: 77%; Protein: 16%; Carbs: 7%

1. Preheat the oven to 375°F.
2. Put the zucchini in a large bowl and sprinkle with the salt. Toss well and set aside.
3. Melt the butter in a small saucepan over medium-low heat. Add the garlic and cook, stirring frequently, until fragrant, about 2 minutes. Set aside.
4. In a medium saucepan over medium heat, melt together the cream cheese, ⅓ cup of mozzarella, and the Brie. Stir frequently until combined. Reduce the heat to low.
5. Stir in the cream, garlic, Italian seasoning, pepper, and nutmeg until completely incorporated.
6. Spray a pie pan or baking dish with cooking spray. Alternate layers of zucchini and cheese mixture in the pan, starting with a third of zucchini topped with a third of the cheese mixture. Repeat twice more. Sprinkle the remaining ⅓ cup of mozzarella on top.
7. Bake for 40 to 45 minutes, until the cheese is golden brown. Serve immediately or cool to room temperature before covering with plastic wrap and refrigerating for up to 4 days.

Creamy Green Bean Casserole

SERVES 6 | PREP TIME: 10 MINUTES | COOK TIME: 40 MINUTES

Most often associated with Thanksgiving, a green bean casserole gives mashed potatoes a run for their money as the favorite holiday side dish. The traditional recipe uses condensed cream of mushroom soup. This recipe makes its own creamy mushroom sauce and is finished with a crunchy, savory pork-rind topping.

2 tablespoons butter

1 cup sliced mushroom caps (such as shiitake)

¼ cup diced white onions

4 ounces full-fat cream cheese, at room temperature

½ cup heavy cream

¼ cup grated parmesan cheese

¼ teaspoon salt

⅛ teaspoon freshly ground black pepper

⅛ teaspoon allspice

2 (14.5 ounce) cans green beans, drained

¾ cup crushed pork rinds

½ cup shredded cheddar cheese

Per Serving (⅔ cup): Calories: 266; Total fat: 23g; Total carbs: 7g; Fiber: 2g; Net carbs: 5g; Protein: 9g; Macronutrients: Fat: 77%; Protein: 13%; Carbs: 10%

1. Preheat the oven to 350°F.
2. Melt the butter in a large saucepan over medium heat. Turn the heat up to medium high and add the mushrooms. Cook for about 5 minutes, until the mushrooms begin to brown.
3. Lower the heat to medium. Add the onions and cook, stirring frequently, until translucent, 3 to 4 minutes.
4. Lower the heat to medium-low and stir in the cream cheese until melted and fully incorporated. Slowly whisk in the cream and parmesan.
5. Stir in the salt, pepper, and allspice. Add the beans and stir until completely coated.
6. Pour the mixture into an 8-by-8-inch baking dish. Top with the pork rinds and cheddar.
7. Bake for 25 to 30 minutes, until the cheese is bubbly and lightly browned. Serve immediately or refrigerate for up to 3 days.

Brussels Sprouts and Bacon

SERVES 4 | PREP TIME: 10 MINUTES | COOK TIME: 40 MINUTES

When I was a child, I loathed Brussels sprouts. My mom would buy them frozen and heat them into some sort of sour mush pile. As it turns out, I actually love them when they are crispy and flavorful. Similar to a smashed potato, these Brussels are crispy on the outside and soft in the middle. With smoky bacon and melted cheese, this recipe makes a warm, flavorful side dish or appetizer.

4 cups water
1 teaspoon sea salt, divided
1 pound Brussels sprouts, trimmed
1 tablespoon olive oil
¼ teaspoon garlic powder
⅛ teaspoon freshly ground black pepper
½ cup grated parmesan cheese
4 slices raw bacon, chopped

Per Serving (¼ recipe):
Calories: 169; Total fat: 10g; Total carbs: 12g; Fiber: 4g; Net carbs: 8g; Protein: 10g; Macronutrients: Fat: 53%; Protein: 21%; Carbs: 26%

1. Preheat the oven to 425°F. Line a baking sheet with parchment paper.
2. Bring the water and ½ teaspoon of salt to a boil in a large saucepan over high heat.
3. Add the sprouts and cook for 10 minutes. Drain and transfer them to a large bowl.
4. Sprinkle them with the remaining ½ teaspoon of salt, the olive oil, the garlic powder, and the pepper and toss to coat.
5. Pour the sprouts onto the prepared baking sheet. Using the bottom of a mug or glass, smash them.
6. Bake for 7 minutes. Remove from the oven, evenly sprinkle with the parmesan and bacon, and bake for another 13 minutes or until the bacon is crisp. Serve immediately or refrigerate for up to 4 days.

SUBSTITUTION TIP: This recipe works well with most cheeses, as long as they melt and crisp. Try shredded cheddar, gouda, or pepper Jack.

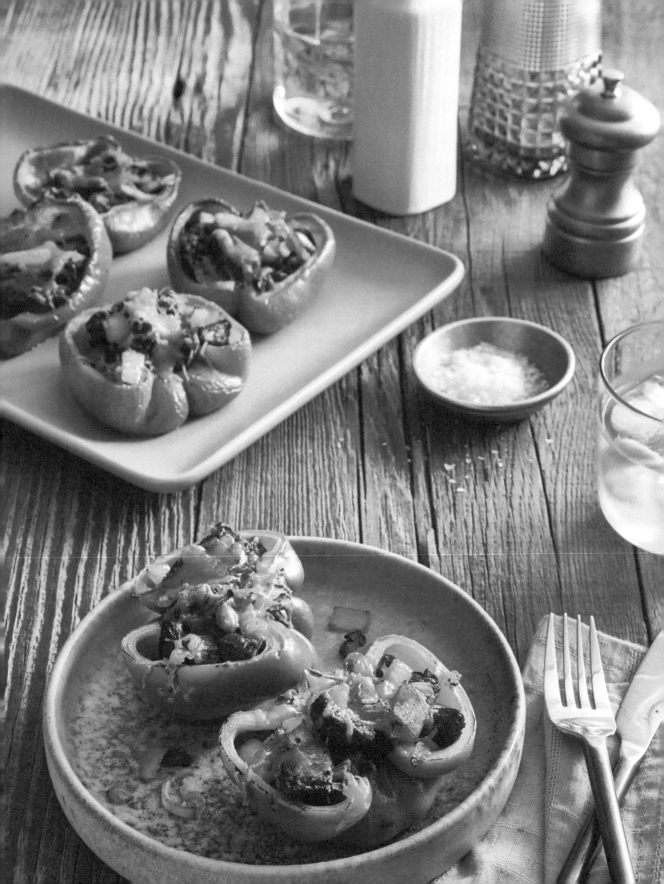

Cheesesteak-Stuffed Peppers

SERVES 4 | PREP TIME: 15 MINUTES | COOK TIME: 40 MINUTES

For those visiting my old hometown of Philadelphia, PA, the proper way to order a cheesesteak is asking for it "wiz wit"—a mixture of Cheez Whiz and onions. This recipe trades the roll for green bell peppers and adds fatty, flavorful skirt steak.

Cooking spray
1¼ teaspoons sea
  salt, divided
4 medium green bell
  peppers, halved
  lengthwise, seeded
2 tablespoons olive
  oil, divided
1 pound skirt steak,
  thinly sliced
½ cup sliced white onions
¼ teaspoon freshly ground
  black pepper
1 cup shredded
  cheddar cheese

Per Serving (1 stuffed pepper): Calories: 487; Total fat: 33g; Total carbs: 9g; Fiber: 2g; Net carbs: 7g; Protein: 39g; Macronutrients: Fat: 61%; Protein: 33%; Carbs: 6%

1. Preheat the oven to 400°F. Spray a baking dish with cooking spray.

2. Sprinkle ¼ teaspoon of salt into the cavity of each pepper half. Place the peppers cut-side up in the baking dish and bake for 15 to 20 minutes, until soft.

3. Meanwhile, heat 1 tablespoon of olive oil in a large skillet over medium-high heat. Add the steak and cook, stirring frequently, until cooked through, about 6 minutes. Transfer to a dish or bowl and set aside.

4. In the same skillet over medium heat, add the remaining 1 tablespoon of olive oil and stir in the onions. Cook until translucent, about 5 minutes.

5. Return the steak to the skillet, season with the remaining 1 teaspoon of salt and the pepper and cook for 1 more minute.

6. Spoon the steak and onion mixture equally inside each pepper half. Top equally with the cheddar. Bake for 3 to 5 minutes, until the cheese melts and begins to brown. Serve immediately or refrigerate for up to 3 days.

PREPARATION TIP: Add ⅓ cup thinly sliced white mushroom caps for vitamin D and flavor. Cook the mushrooms with the onions, but add 5 to 7 minutes to the cooking time so the juice from the mushrooms evaporates.

Prosciutto-Wrapped Asparagus

SERVES 4 | PREP TIME: 15 MINUTES | COOK TIME: 15 MINUTES

Prosciutto-wrapped asparagus is not just for party appetizers; it also makes a great entrée. Melted cheese and savory pork envelop a crisp, fresh asparagus spear. Roasting asparagus in olive oil gives this vegetable dish sweet notes, making it a nice complement to eggs for an upgraded and comforting brunch. Try it with a side of hollandaise (see Easy Eggs Benedict, page 27) for a rich, creamy bite.

16 thin slices prosciutto
16 thin slices
 provolone cheese
16 thick asparagus spears,
 woody ends trimmed
½ tablespoon olive oil
⅛ teaspoon freshly
 ground black pepper

Per Serving (4 wrapped asparagus): Calories: 395; Total fat: 28g; Total carbs: 6g; Fiber: 2g; Net carbs: 4g; Protein: 32g; Macronutrients: Fat: 61%; Protein: 34%; Carbs: 5%

1. Preheat the oven to 425°F. Line a baking sheet with parchment paper.
2. On the baking sheet, lay 1 piece of prosciutto, then top it with 1 provolone slice. Lay 1 asparagus spear on the far side of the cheese and then roll it in the prosciutto and provolone. Repeat with the remaining slices and spears.
3. Lay the wrapped asparagus in a single layer on the prepared baking sheet. Drizzle with the olive oil and sprinkle evenly with pepper.
4. Bake for 8 to 12 minutes, until the asparagus is fork-tender and the cheese underneath bubbles out. Serve immediately or refrigerate in a single layer for up to 4 days.

SUBSTITUTION TIP: Sprinkle about ¼ teaspoon each ground hazelnuts and lemon zest on top of each asparagus spear before rolling them up.

Sausage-Stuffed Mushrooms

SERVES 4 | PREP TIME: 15 MINUTES | COOK TIME: 40 MINUTES

Could you create a filling, comforting meal out of vegetables and meat alone? If my meal included Sausage-Stuffed Mushrooms, I surely could. Choose large mushrooms, such as portobello, for this recipe to ensure you get more cheesy sausage filling in each bite.

6 ounces ground
  Italian sausage
¼ cup diced white onion
1 garlic clove, minced
2 ounces full-fat
  cream cheese, at
  room temperature
¼ cup grated
  parmesan cheese
12 baby portobello
  mushrooms, cleaned
  and stemmed
⅓ cup shredded
  mozzarella cheese

Per Serving (3 stuffed mushrooms): Calories: 269; Total fat: 20g; Total carbs: 8g; Fiber: 1g; Net carbs: 7g; Protein: 15g; Macronutrients: Fat: 67%; Protein: 22%; Carbs: 11%

1. Preheat the oven to 375°F. Line a baking sheet with parchment paper.
2. Heat a large frying pan over medium heat. Add the sausage and cook, breaking the meat into small pieces, until browned, about 5 minutes. Use a slotted spoon to transfer the meat to a bowl, leaving the fat.
3. In the same pan over medium heat, cook the onion and garlic until softened, about 5 more minutes.
4. Return the sausage to the pan and stir in the cream cheese and parmesan. Continue to stir until the cream cheese has melted.
5. Spoon the mixture evenly into each mushroom cap. Top equally with the mozzarella.
6. Bake for 20 to 25 minutes, until the mushrooms are soft and the cheese bubbles.
7. Serve immediately or refrigerate for up to 2 days.

> **PREPARATION TIP:** As a way to ensure that your mushrooms don't get too watery before baking, sprinkle them with a little salt and let them sit while you're making the filling. The salt will draw the moisture out.

Bacon-Wrapped Onion Rings

SERVES 4 | PREP TIME: 20 MINUTES | COOK TIME: 30 MINUTES

When you simply need a crunchy onion ring without the extra carbs—or mess from deep-frying—make this recipe. Baked and served with a spicy-smoky dip, these onion rings are an easy-to-clean-up, crispy, comforting snack.

1 medium white onion, cut into 8 rounds
16 slices sugar-free bacon
¼ cup avocado oil mayonnaise
2 teaspoons hot sauce
¼ teaspoon sea salt
¼ teaspoon paprika
⅛ teaspoon freshly ground black pepper

Per Serving (2 onion rings):
Calories: 354; Total fat: 32g;
Total carbs: 3g; Fiber: 1g;
Net carbs: 2g; Protein: 16g;
Macronutrients: Fat: 78%;
Protein: 18%; Carbs: 4%

1. Preheat the oven to 375°F. Line a baking sheet with parchment paper. Line a plate with paper towels.
2. Remove 3 inner layers of each onion slice to form rings. Store the unused layers for later use.
3. Starting from the inside, wrap 2 slices of bacon around each onion ring.
4. Lay the rings in a single layer on the prepared baking sheet. Bake for 15 minutes. Flip and bake for another 10 to 12 minutes, until the bacon is cooked through.
5. Transfer the onion rings to the prepared plate to crisp.
6. In a small bowl, whisk together the mayonnaise, hot sauce, salt, paprika, and pepper.
7. Serve the onion rings with the mayonnaise sauce for dipping. Refrigerate leftovers for up to 2 days and reheat under the broiler for 1 to 2 minutes to crisp.

Coleslaw

SERVES 6 | PREP TIME: 1 HOUR 10 MINUTES

I turned my nose up at coleslaw as a child. These days, I enjoy this crunchy salad on its own, as a filling side dish, or as a crispy topper for keto-friendly sandwiches. With its creamy mix of avocado oil mayonnaise and tang of vinegar and mustard, this coleslaw is a vegetable dish I crave.

½ cup avocado
  oil mayonnaise
1 tablespoon erythritol
2 tablespoons lemon juice
2 tablespoons apple
  cider vinegar
½ teaspoon Dijon mustard
½ teaspoon sea salt
¼ teaspoon garlic powder
¼ teaspoon freshly ground
  black pepper
2 cups bagged
  coleslaw mix

Per Serving (⅔ cup): Calories: 142; Total fat: 16g; Total carbs: 6g; Fiber: 1g; Net carbs: 5g; Protein: <1g; Macronutrients: Fat: 95%; Protein: 1%; Carbs: 4%

1. In a large bowl, whisk together all ingredients with the exception of the coleslaw mix until well combined.
2. Stir in the coleslaw mix until the vegetables are completely coated in the dressing.
3. Cover and refrigerate for 1 hour.
4. Serve, or transfer to an airtight container and refrigerate for up to 3 days.

FEEDING THE FAMILY: Consider adding broccoli or cauliflower florets, shredded cheddar cheese, cooked and crumbled bacon, or sunflower seeds for a more robust side dish.

Creamed Spinach

Spinach is a popular vegetable in the keto community because it's low-carb and nutrient rich. This dish is extra creamy, thanks to the cream, tangy cream cheese, and savory parmesan. It is a delicious side for any meal. My favorite way to enjoy this dish is serving it between Canadian bacon and eggs in Easy Eggs Benedict (page 27).

1 tablespoon butter
¼ cup diced white onion
1 garlic clove, minced
10 ounces chopped frozen spinach, thawed and well drained
¼ cup heavy cream
2 ounces full-fat cream cheese, at room temperature
¼ cup grated parmesan cheese
½ teaspoon salt
⅛ teaspoon freshly ground black pepper
Pinch nutmeg

Per Serving (⅓ recipe): Calories: 238; Total fat: 20g; Total carbs: 9g; Fiber: 3g; Net carbs: 6g; Protein: 8g; Macronutrients: Fat: 75%; Protein: 11%; Carbs: 14%

1. Melt the butter in a medium frying pan over medium heat. Add the onion and cook for 3 minutes, stirring frequently. Add the garlic and cook until fragrant, about 1 more minute.

2. Stir in the spinach and cook for 4 to 5 minutes, until any residual water from the spinach evaporates.

3. Slowly stir in the cream. Drop the heat to medium low and stir in the cream cheese. Keep stirring until the cream cheese has melted.

4. Stir in the parmesan, salt, pepper, and nutmeg until completely combined.

5. Serve immediately or refrigerate for up to 4 days.

MAKE IT DAIRY-FREE: Substitute thick, canned coconut milk for the heavy cream, almond or cashew cream "cheese" for the dairy cream cheese, and omit the parmesan.

Broccoli Cheese Casserole

SERVES 4 | PREP TIME: 10 MINUTES | COOK TIME: 20 MINUTES

Smothered in cheese sauce is one way to get even the pickiest eater to enjoy their vegetables. This casserole can be served as a side dish or made with a protein for a well-rounded comfort food meal.

Cooking spray
2 cups fresh
  broccoli florets
2 tablespoons water
¼ cup avocado oil
  mayonnaise
¼ cup full-fat sour cream
1 teaspoon Dijon mustard
¾ teaspoon sea salt
½ teaspoon garlic powder
⅛ teaspoon freshly ground
  black pepper
1¼ cups shredded cheddar
  cheese, divided

Per Serving (½ cup): Calories: 281; Total fat: 26g; Total carbs: 4g; Fiber: 1g; Net carbs: 3g; Protein: 10g; Macronutrients: Fat: 80%; Protein: 14%; Carbs: 6%

1. Preheat the oven to 375°F. Spray an 8-by-8-inch baking dish with cooking spray.
2. Place the broccoli and water in a microwave-safe bowl. Cover and microwave on high for 3 minutes. Set aside but leave the bowl covered.
3. In a large bowl, whisk together the mayonnaise, sour cream, Dijon, salt, garlic powder, and pepper until well combined. Stir in ¾ cup of cheddar.
4. Drain the broccoli and stir it into the mayo-cheese mixture until the broccoli is completely coated.
5. Pour the broccoli mixture into the prepared dish. Top evenly with the remaining ½ cup of cheddar.
6. Bake for 15 minutes. Remove and turn the oven to broil. Broil the casserole for 2 to 3 minutes, until the top layer of cheese is lightly browned and bubbly. Serve immediately or allow the casserole to come to room temperature before covering and refrigerating for up to 4 days.

> **FEEDING THE FAMILY:** Cooked, shredded chicken, ground turkey, and bacon are all tasty additions. Incorporate the protein in step 4 and then follow the remaining directions.

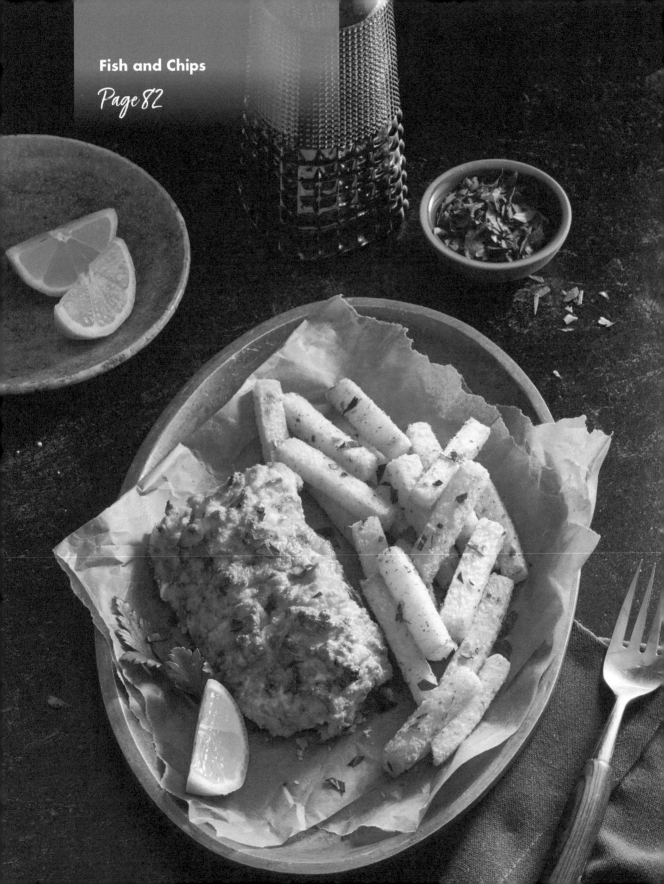

Fish and Chips

Page 82

Chapter 5

FISH AND SEAFOOD

Glazed Salmon

SERVES 4 | PREP TIME: 10 MINUTES | COOK TIME: 15 MINUTES

Growing up, I thought I didn't like fish because it tasted "too fishy." This was before I tasted salmon. Packed with protein, vitamins, minerals, and an abundance of omega-3 fatty acids, salmon is one of the most keto-friendly fish. Coated with a maple glaze and tangy Dijon mustard, it might be easy to forget how healthy this salmon dish truly is.

Cooking spray

2 tablespoons sugar-free maple syrup

2 tablespoons Dijon mustard

2 teaspoons melted coconut oil

4 (6-ounce) skinless salmon fillets, rinsed and patted dry

1 teaspoon sea salt

¼ teaspoon freshly ground black pepper

Per Serving (1 fillet): Calories: 230; Total fat: 9g; Total carbs: 2g; Fiber: 2g; Net carbs: 0g; Protein: 33g; Macronutrients: Fat: 60%; Protein: 37%; Carbs: 3%

1. Preheat oven to 400°F. Line a baking sheet with aluminum foil and lightly spray with cooking spray.
2. In a small bowl, whisk together the sugar-free maple syrup, mustard, and coconut oil.
3. Season the salmon with the salt and pepper. Spoon half the sauce evenly over each fillet. Place the salmon skin-side down on the foil.
4. Bake for 8 minutes. Spoon the remaining sauce evenly over each fillet, and then bake for another 3 to 4 minutes or until the fish flakes easily.
5. Serve immediately or refrigerate for up to 2 days.

PREPARATION TIP: Be sure to buy skinned salmon, or remove the skin before it goes in the oven. Roasted salmon skin will never crisp and will instead become gummy.

Tuna Melt

SERVES 2 | PREP TIME: 10 MINUTES | COOK TIME: 5 MINUTES

Second only to a BLT, a tuna melt is my go-to sandwich when I am looking to bite into some comfort. A tuna melt is basically the marriage of tuna salad and a grilled cheese sandwich. The toasted 90-Second Bread and celery provide a playful crunch to the soft sandwich interior. Easy to prep and easy to cook, this recipe can be enjoyed even on the busiest of days.

2 batches 90-Second Bread (page 158; see Note)

2 (6-ounce) cans solid white albacore tuna in water, drained

¼ cup plus 2 tablespoons avocado oil mayonnaise

1 tablespoon Dijon mustard

1 celery stalk, diced

1 teaspoon freshly squeezed lemon juice

¼ teaspoon dried parsley

⅛ teaspoon freshly ground black pepper

4 slices cheddar cheese

Per Serving (½ recipe): Calories: 936; Total fat: 82g; Total carbs: 6g; Fiber: 3g; Net carbs: 3g; Protein: 52g; Macronutrients: Fat: 75%; Protein: 23%; Carbs: 2%

1. Preheat the oven to broil. Line a baking sheet with parchment paper.
2. In a medium bowl, mix together the tuna, mayonnaise, mustard, celery, lemon juice, parsley, and pepper. Stir until thoroughly combined.
3. Make the 90-Second Bread. When each piece is cool enough to handle, slice in half and toast.
4. Lay the 4 pieces of toast on the prepared baking sheet. Top each piece with an equal amount of tuna salad, followed by a slice of cheese.
5. Broil for 2 to 3 minutes or until the cheese has melted. Serve immediately. This dish does not store well, so halve the recipe if needed.

NOTE: Make the 90-Second Bread with 1 tablespoon olive oil in lieu of the butter.

PREPARATION TIP: Adding veggies such as cooked spinach and a slice of tomato ups the flavor, texture, and nutrition for this tuna melt. Top the tuna salad with your vegetables of choice, and then top with the cheese before broiling.

Tuna Casserole

SERVES 6 | PREP TIME: 20 MINUTES | COOK TIME: 40 MINUTES

As a child, I went grocery shopping with my mom, and we bought a box mix for tuna noodle casserole. All you had to do was add tuna. We made it, and it was pretty awful. Not until I made my own from scratch did I jump back on the tuna noodle casserole fan wagon. When making this recipe, be sure to squeeze out excess water from the zoodles to avoid a watery dish.

3 cups Zoodles (page 166)
1½ teaspoons salt, divided
Cooking spray
1 tablespoon avocado oil
¼ cup diced white onion
½ cup thinly sliced
   baby portobello
   mushroom caps
1 garlic clove, minced
¼ teaspoon freshly
   ground black pepper
2 (6-ounce) cans solid
   white albacore tuna in
   water, drained
½ cup avocado
   oil mayonnaise
2 teaspoons Dijon mustard
1 teaspoon freshly
   squeezed lemon juice
½ cup shredded
   cheddar cheese
½ cup shredded
   mozzarella cheese

Per Serving (⅙ of recipe):
Calories: 310; Total fat: 26g;
Total carbs: 7g; Fiber: 2g;
Net carbs: 5g; Protein: 17g;
Macronutrients: Fat: 71%;
Protein: 21%; Carbs: 8%

1. Lay paper towels on top of a baking sheet. Spread the zoodles onto the paper towels, sprinkle with 1 teaspoon salt, and cover with another layer of paper towels. Lightly press down on the zoodles to draw out the water. Allow the zoodles to sit, covered in paper towels, and set aside.

2. Preheat the oven to 350°F. Spray a 9-by-13-inch casserole dish with cooking spray.

3. In a large skillet over medium heat, warm the avocado oil. Add the onion and mushrooms and cook, stirring frequently, for 4 to 5 minutes or until the onion becomes translucent and the mushrooms begin to brown.

4. Stir in the garlic and cook for 1 more minute.

5. Add the zoodles, remaining ½ teaspoon of salt, and the pepper. Cook, stirring frequently, for about 3 more minutes. The zoodles should be cooked but still al dente. Remove from the heat.

6. In a large bowl, use a fork to mix together the tuna, mayonnaise, mustard, and lemon juice until well combined.

7. Add the cooked vegetables and stir to coat everything in the tuna mixture.

8. Pour the mixture into the prepared dish. Cover with the cheddar and mozzarella.

9. Bake for 25 to 30 minutes or until the cheese is golden and bubbly.

10. Let the casserole sit for 2 to 3 minutes. Serve immediately or refrigerate for up to 2 days.

SUBSTITUTION TIP: Not a fan of tuna? Shredded or canned chicken or cooked ground turkey can replace it.

Fish Tacos

SERVES 4 | PREP TIME: 15 MINUTES | COOK TIME: 20 MINUTES

Both filling and light, fish tacos are served everywhere from hole-in-the-wall beach shacks to fine dining establishments. In this recipe, we lean on butter lettuce's freshness and coleslaw's creaminess to enhance the battered cod's crunch. Go as spicy as you wish to make this recipe your own. If cod is not available, any white fish works well.

1 large egg, beaten
½ cup coconut flour, divided
1 teaspoon salt
1 teaspoon ground cumin
¼ teaspoon paprika
⅛ teaspoon chili powder
1 pound skinless boneless cod, cut into 1-inch pieces, patted dry
8 large butter lettuce leaves
½ recipe Coleslaw (page 71)
1 sliced avocado
¼ cup pico de gallo, divided
1 quartered lime

Per Serving (2 tacos): Calories: 344; Total fat: 22g; Total carbs: 19g; Fiber: 9g; Net carbs: 10g; Protein: 25g; Macronutrients: Fat: 57%; Protein: 29%; Carbs: 14%

1. Preheat the oven to 400°F. Line a baking sheet with parchment paper.
2. Pour the egg into a small bowl. Pour ¼ cup of coconut flour into a medium bowl. In a second medium bowl, thoroughly combine the remaining ¼ cup of coconut flour, salt, cumin, paprika, and chili powder.
3. Dip the cod pieces first into the plain coconut flour, then the egg, and finally the seasoned flour.
4. Lay the cod on the prepared baking sheet in a single layer. Bake for 10 minutes, flip, and then bake for another 10 minutes. Let cool for 2 minutes.
5. To assemble the tacos, lay out the lettuce leaves and top with equal amounts of cod, coleslaw, avocado, and pico de gallo. Squeeze lime juice on top. Serve immediately.

Crab Cakes

SERVES 6 | PREP TIME: 25 MINUTES | COOK TIME: 10 MINUTES

Crab meat is naturally soft and buttery, like a little seafood pillow. It doesn't take many ingredients to make a crab cake delicious. These crab cakes take a little care to make them light and airy; be gentle when combining the ingredients to keep the succulent jumbo lump crab meat intact.

1 large egg, separated
½ cup avocado oil mayonnaise
1 tablespoon Dijon mustard
1 teaspoon Old Bay seasoning (see tip for substitute)
1 teaspoon dried parsley
1 pound jumbo lump crab meat, picked over for shell pieces
⅓ cup crushed pork rinds
2 tablespoons avocado oil, divided
Lemon wedges, for serving (optional)

Per Serving (1 crab cake): Calories: 262; Total fat: 23g; Total carbs: <1g; Fiber: <1g; Net carbs: <1g; Protein: 16g; Macronutrients: Fat: 74%; Protein: 26%; Carbs: <1%

1. Line a baking sheet with parchment paper.
2. In a large bowl, whisk together the egg yolk, mayonnaise, mustard, Old Bay seasoning, and parsley until well combined. Gently fold in the crab, being careful to leave large lumps of crab meat.
3. In a second large bowl, beat the egg white until soft peaks form. Gently fold the egg whites into the crab mixture, keeping as many large lumps of crab meat as possible. Gently fold in the pork rinds.
4. Divide the crab mixture into 6 equal portions and form into patties. Place the patties on the prepared baking sheet and refrigerate for 15 minutes.
5. Heat 1 tablespoon of avocado oil in a large skillet over medium heat. Place 3 crab cakes in the skillet and cook for 3 to 4 minutes per side, just until golden and cooked through. Repeat with the remaining tablespoon of avocado oil and 3 crab cakes.
6. Serve immediately with lemon wedges (if using).

> **SUBSTITUTION TIP:** If you do not have Old Bay seasoning, combine ½ teaspoon paprika, ¼ teaspoon sea salt, and ⅛ teaspoon each cayenne pepper and black pepper.

Fish and Chips

SERVES | PREP TIME: 45 MINUTES | COOK TIME: 1 HOUR

I fell in love with fish and chips while waiting tables at an Irish pub. The deep-fried fish had me at the accompaniment of a platter of fries. Instead of battering our fish in flour and deep-frying them in oil, this recipe creates a light, crunchy, gluten-free batter with the help of club soda. We bake instead of fry, simplifying the cooking and cleanup.

1½ tablespoons butter, melted

1 large egg, beaten

½ cup coconut flour, divided

¼ cup crushed pork rinds

½ teaspoon freshly ground black pepper

1½ teaspoons dried parsley

1 cup almond flour

1 teaspoon baking powder

½ teaspoon sea salt

1 (12-ounce) can club soda

4 (6-ounce) cod fillets, patted dry

Lemon wedges (optional)

1 batch Jicama Fries (page 61)

Per Serving (1 fillet and ½ cup fries): Calories: 492; Total fat: 30g; Total carbs: 17g; Fiber: 9g; Net carbs: 8g; Protein: 41g; Macronutrients: Fat: 55%; Protein: 33%; Carbs: 12%

1. Preheat the oven to 450°F.
2. Pour the butter into a rimmed baking dish, spreading it evenly.
3. Pour the egg into a small bowl. In a medium bowl, thoroughly combine ¼ cup of coconut flour, pork rinds, pepper, and parsley. In a second medium bowl, thoroughly combine the almond flour, baking powder, remaining ¼ cup of coconut flour, and salt.
4. Slowly whisk the club soda into the flour mixture until it resembles thin pancake batter.
5. Dredge the cod fillets first in the coconut–pork rind mixture, then the egg, and finally the almond flour batter.

6. Place the fillets in the baking dish and bake for 20 minutes or until golden brown (watch to avoid burning). To brown them further (which I highly recommend), broil for an additional 5 minutes. Serve immediately with lemon wedges (if using) and fries.

> **PREPARATION TIP:** Hold off on mixing the almond flour–club soda batter until you are ready to dip the fish. This way the consistency will stay liquid enough to prevent clumping. If the batter does begin to clump, simply use a spoon to cover the fillet in batter. Frozen cod also works here; just be sure to thaw it completely first.

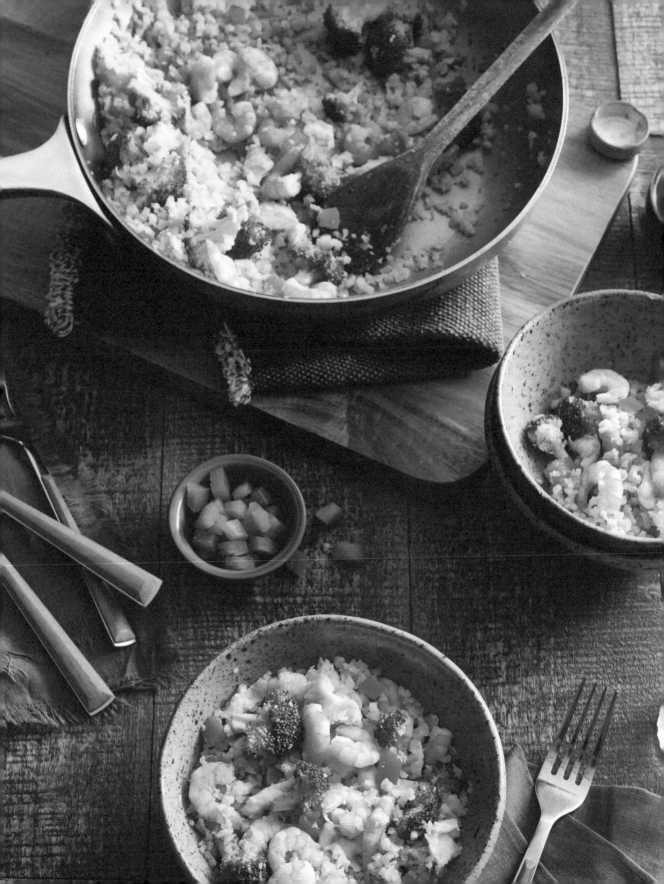

Shrimp Fried Rice

SERVES 4 | PREP TIME: 20 MINUTES | COOK TIME: 15 MINUTES

When we ordered Chinese takeout in college, not all my roommates could agree on what to share—except shrimp fried rice. This recipe uses caulirice to keep the carbs low. If you cannot find coconut aminos, feel free to use your favorite brand of low-sodium soy sauce.

2 tablespoons coconut oil, divided
1 pound peeled and deveined shrimp
½ teaspoon sea salt
⅛ teaspoon freshly ground black pepper
3 cups Caulirice (page 163)
¼ cup diced red bell pepper
¼ cup chopped broccoli florets
2 tablespoons diced white onion
2 garlic cloves, minced
2 large eggs
2 tablespoons coconut aminos

Per Serving (¼ recipe): Calories: 217; Total fat: 12g; Total carbs: 10g; Fiber: 2g; Net carbs: 8g; Protein: 20g; Macronutrients: Fat: 49%; Protein: 37%; Carbs: 14%

1. Heat 1 tablespoon of oil in a large skillet over high heat.
2. Add the shrimp and season with the salt and pepper. Sauté the shrimp until pink, about 3 minutes. Transfer to a plate and set aside.
3. In the same skillet over medium-high heat, heat the remaining 1 tablespoon of oil. Add the caulirice and cook, stirring frequently, until most of its water has evaporated, 5 to 7 minutes.
4. Stir in the bell pepper, broccoli, and onion. Cook, stirring frequently, until the onions are translucent, about 3 minutes. Stir in the garlic and cook for 1 more minute.
5. Move the veggies toward the outer edges of the skillet. Crack the eggs into the middle of the pan and allow to cook untouched for 1 minute.
6. Mix the veggies into the egg, scrambling the egg as you go. Cook for another minute, until the eggs are cooked through.
7. Add the shrimp and coconut aminos. Stir thoroughly to fully incorporate. Serve, or refrigerate overnight.

FEEDING THE FAMILY: Fried rice is an adaptable dish that supports the addition of more low-carb vegetables, such as cauliflower and mushrooms, as well as different proteins.

Shrimp Scampi

SERVES 4 | PREP TIME: 20 MINUTES | COOK TIME: 15 MINUTES

Succulent shrimp swimming in an entire stick of melted butter and fragrant garlic, shrimp scampi is a quick and easy Italian American comfort food recipe. Fresh zoodles cooked al dente soak up the buttery sauce while keeping this dish low-carb and keto-friendly. Add more red pepper flakes for extra heat or omit them completely for a milder dish.

2 cups Zoodles (page 166)
1½ teaspoons sea
  salt, divided
½ cup (1 stick) unsalted
  butter, cut into cubes
4 garlic cloves, minced
¼ teaspoon red
  pepper flakes
1 pound medium peeled
  and deveined shrimp
⅛ teaspoon freshly ground
  black pepper
1 tablespoon freshly
  squeezed lemon juice
2 teaspoons dried parsley
2 tablespoons
  parmesan cheese

Per Serving (¼ recipe):
Calories: 330; Total fat: 25g;
Total carbs: 7g; Fiber: 2;
Net carbs: 5g; Protein: 20g;
Macronutrients: Fat: 68%;
Protein: 25%; Carbs: 7%

1. Line a baking sheet with paper towels. Spread the zoodles on the paper towels, sprinkle with 1 teaspoon of salt, and cover with another layer of paper towels. Lightly press to absorb water. Set aside.
2. Melt the butter in a large skillet over medium heat. Add the garlic and red pepper flakes and cook, stirring frequently, until fragrant, about 2 minutes.
3. Add the shrimp. Season with the remaining ½ teaspoon of salt and the black pepper. Cook for 2 minutes, just until the shrimp are pink.
4. Stir in the zoodles and lemon juice until well combined. Sprinkle with the parsley and stir again.
5. Serve immediately, topped with the parmesan, or refrigerate for up to 2 days.

SUBSTITUTION TIP: Boneless skinless chicken thighs can replace the shrimp. Cut the chicken into 1-inch pieces and cook in 2 tablespoons of melted butter over medium-high heat for about 5 minutes per side or until cooked through. Set aside, and then follow the recipe steps from the beginning.

Popcorn Shrimp

SERVES 2 | PREP TIME: 15 MINUTES | COOK TIME: 8 MINUTES

Crispy, flavorful, and quick to cook, popcorn shrimp can be eaten by the handful and served in a variety of ways, such as with a side of your favorite vegetables for a complete meal or in fish tacos. You can even make a filling po' boy sandwich by layering the crispy baked shrimp, crisp lettuce, a slice of fresh tomato, and avocado oil mayonnaise between two pieces of toasted 90-Second Bread (page 158).

½ cup coconut oil
2 large eggs
1 crushed chicken
   bouillon cube
⅓ cup coconut flour
½ teaspoon chili
   powder (optional)
½ pound small peeled,
   deveined shrimp

Per Serving (½ recipe):
Calories: 452; Total fat: 35g;
Total carbs: 12g; Fiber: 7g;
Net carbs: 5g; Protein: 22g;
Macronutrients: Fat: 70%;
Protein: 19%; Carbs: 11%

1. Line a plate with paper towels.
2. Melt the oil in a medium saucepan over medium heat. The oil should be ½ inch deep.
3. In a large bowl, beat the eggs. In another large bowl, whisk together the bouillon cube, coconut flour, and chili powder (if using).
4. Drop ¼ cup of shrimp at a time first into the eggs and then the flour mixture until each shrimp is completely coated.
5. Add the coated shrimp, ¼ cup at a time, to the oil, making sure each shrimp is submerged in the oil (adding more oil if necessary). Fry until golden, about 2 minutes per side.
6. Use a slotted spoon to transfer the fried shrimp to the prepared plate. Repeat with the remaining shrimp, cooking in ¼-cup batches. Serve immediately.

Shrimp and Grits

SERVES 4 | PREP TIME: 20 MINUTES | COOK TIME: 25 MINUTES

The first time I ordered shrimp and grits at a Southern restaurant, I practically licked my bowl clean. Smoky bacon, butter, cream, and cheese transform low-carb caulirice into a bowl of rich, cozy, keto-friendly comfort.

1 pound medium peeled, deveined shrimp
1 teaspoon salt, divided
¼ teaspoon freshly ground black pepper, divided
⅛ teaspoon chili powder
4 slices bacon
2 tablespoons butter
3 cups Caulirice (page 163)
½ cup shredded cheddar
¼ cup shredded parmesan cheese
½ cup heavy cream
2 thinly sliced small scallions

Per Serving (¼ recipe): Calories: 369; Total fat: 26g; Total carbs: 6g; Fiber: 2g; Net carbs: 4g; Protein: 28g; Macronutrients: Fat: 63%; Protein: 30%; Carbs: 7%

1. Line two plates with paper towels.
2. In a large bowl, toss together the shrimp, ½ teaspoon of salt, ⅛ teaspoon of pepper, and the chili powder. Cover and refrigerate.
3. In a large skillet over medium heat, fry the bacon until crisp. Transfer to one of the prepared plates. Set the skillet aside, reserving 2 tablespoons of grease.
4. In a medium saucepan on medium-low heat, melt the butter. Add the caulirice and stir to coat. Cook for 3 minutes, stirring frequently.
5. Slowly stir in the cheddar and parmesan until well combined. Next, stir in the cream and remaining salt and pepper.
6. Increase the heat to medium high and simmer, stirring frequently, until the rice becomes soft and smooth, about 10 minutes.
7. Heat the reserved bacon grease in the skillet over medium heat. Add the shrimp and sauté until pink and cooked through, 3 to 5 minutes. Use a slotted spoon to transfer the shrimp to the second prepared plate.
8. Serve the caulirice mixture in bowls, topped with the shrimp, crumbled bacon, and scallions.

MAKE AHEAD: Make the grits the day before. Reheat on the stovetop over medium-low heat for 3 to 5 minutes.

Buffalo Wings

Page 99

Chapter 6

POULTRY

Whole Roasted Chicken

SERVES 6 | PREP TIME: 30 MINUTES | COOK TIME: 1 HOUR 15 MINUTES

Before graduating to cooking an entire turkey for Thanksgiving dinner, I cut my teeth on roasting a whole chicken. One of the main issues I had was that the breast would always dry out before the thighs were done cooking. Butter was the game-changer that kept the entire bird juicy.

1 (4- to 5-pound)
  roasting chicken
2 teaspoons sea
  salt, divided
1 teaspoon dried thyme
½ teaspoon freshly ground
  black pepper
1 orange, quartered
2 garlic cloves, minced
3 celery stalks, cut into
  2-inch pieces
1 cup cauliflower florets
1 cup broccoli florets
1 tablespoon avocado oil
4 tablespoons
  salted butter, at
  room temperature
1 teaspoon dried parsley

Per Serving (6 ounces):
Calories: 267; Total fat: 14g;
Total carbs: 6g; Fiber: 2g;
Net carbs: 4g; Protein: 30g;
Macronutrients: Fat: 47%;
Protein: 45%; Carbs: 8%

1. Preheat the oven to 425°F.
2. Remove the giblets from the chicken. Rinse the inside out and pat the outside with the paper towels until it is thoroughly dry.
3. Season the chicken cavity with 1 teaspoon of salt, the thyme, and the pepper. Stuff the cavity with the orange wedges and garlic.
4. Put the celery, cauliflower, and broccoli in a roasting pan. Sprinkle with the remaining 1 teaspoon of salt and cover with the oil.
5. Lay the chicken on top of the vegetables. Massage the butter all over the chicken. Sprinkle evenly with the parsley.
6. Roast for 1 hour and 15 minutes or until the juices run clear when a knife is inserted in the thickest part of the chicken.
7. Let sit for 15 minutes before serving. Refrigerate leftovers for up to 5 days.

> **LOVING YOUR LEFTOVERS:** Serve this chicken as an extra protein in a BLT Sandwich (page 40) with avocado oil mayonnaise and pecans, or swap it for the beef in tacos (page 53).

Crispy Chicken Thighs

SERVES 4 | PREP TIME: 10 MINUTES | COOK TIME: 40 MINUTES

Chicken and mashed potatoes were a staple in my childhood home. We ate frozen chicken breasts and instant mash several times a week. Now that I cook for myself and follow a ketogenic lifestyle, I have transitioned to fresh, crispy, and juicy chicken thighs served with a side of Buttery Caulimash. This meal is a simple classic comfort food dish that comes together in under an hour.

1 teaspoon sea salt
½ teaspoon freshly ground black pepper
½ teaspoon paprika
4 large bone-in, skin-on chicken thighs, patted dry
Baking powder, for dusting (optional)
1 recipe Buttery Caulimash (page 58)

Per Serving (1 thigh + ⅔ cup caulimash): Calories: 423; Total fat: 37g; Total carbs: 4g; Fiber: 2g; Net carbs: 2g; Protein: 22g; Macronutrients: Fat: 79%; Protein: 20%; Carbs: 1%

1. Preheat the oven to 400°F. Line a rimmed baking sheet with parchment paper.
2. In a small bowl, combine the salt, pepper, and paprika. Season each thigh with the spice mix. For extra crispy skin, lightly dust each thigh with a small amount of baking powder.
3. Bake for 40 minutes, until the chicken skin is browned and crisp.
4. Serve the chicken with the caulimash, or refrigerate the chicken and caulimash separately. Chicken thighs will be good for up to 5 days, and caulimash is best within 3 days.

SUBSTITUTION TIP: Although you can use boneless thighs, you'll trade flavor for speed. To help boneless thighs shine, massage ½ tablespoon of softened butter onto the entire thigh before baking for 25 to 30 minutes.

Fried Chicken

SERVES 4 | PREP TIME: 15 MINUTES | COOK TIME: 45 MINUTES

Crispy, crunchy, salty, and juicy, fried chicken is finger-lickin' good. Although a good coating and mix of seasonings play a large role in making fried chicken downright delicious, skin-on chicken is crucial to providing that craveable crunch. Below that salty, fatty bite, bone-in chicken pieces ensure a juicy piece of meat.

3 pounds bone-in, skin-on chicken legs and thighs
2 teaspoons sea salt, divided
2 eggs, beaten
1 teaspoon baking powder
⅓ cup coconut flour
¼ cup almond flour
¼ cup crushed pork rinds
¼ cup grated parmesan cheese (optional)
½ teaspoon garlic powder
½ teaspoon paprika
6 tablespoons unsalted butter, melted

Per Serving (1 piece): Calories: 909; Total fat: 69g; Total carbs: 8g; Fiber: 4g; Net carbs: 4g; Protein: 66g; Macronutrients: Fat: 68%; Protein: 29%; Carbs: 3%

1. Preheat the oven to 425°F. Line a baking pan with aluminum foil. Set a cooking rack in the upper-middle of the oven.
2. Pat the chicken completely dry and season with 1 teaspoon of salt; set aside.
3. Pour the eggs into a small bowl. In a large resealable plastic bag, combine the baking powder and coconut flour. In a second bag, combine the almond flour, pork rinds, parmesan (if using), garlic powder, and paprika.
4. Dredge each piece of chicken first in the coconut flour mixture, then the egg, and then the almond flour mixture, shaking to coat the chicken completely.
5. Pour the butter into the prepared pan, making sure it spreads evenly. Place the chicken parts skin-side down in the pan.

6. Bake for 30 minutes, flip the chicken and rotate the pan, and bake for another 15 to 20 minutes. (If you're using a thermometer, the chicken is done when it reaches an internal temp of 165°F.) Serve immediately or refrigerate for up to 3 days. Reheat under a broiler to crisp up the coating.

> **FEEDING THE FAMILY:** Fried chicken pairs with any vegetable side, but it can also be enjoyed for breakfast and brunch. Serve over Belgian-Style Waffles (page 22) drizzled with sugar-free maple syrup or with a side of Butter Biscuits (page 18).

Chicken Nuggets

MAKES 20 | PREP TIME: 15 MINUTES | COOK TIME: 30 MINUTES

Despite resembling the chicken nuggets from a fast-food restaurant or big frozen bag, these chicken nuggets are a much heartier, healthier version of a childhood favorite. Because this recipe calls for ground chicken, they can take on any form you choose. Dinobites? Shape them using a cookie cutter. Chicken sticks? Whatever comforts your sweet soul.

Cooking spray
1 pound ground chicken
1 large beaten egg
¼ cup almond flour
½ teaspoon sea salt
¼ teaspoon onion powder
⅛ teaspoon freshly ground
   black pepper
¾ cup finely crushed
   pork rinds
3 tablespoons
   parmesan cheese
¾ teaspoon dried oregano
½ teaspoon garlic powder
½ teaspoon paprika

Per Serving (5 nuggets):
Calories: 275; Total fat: 17g;
Total carbs: 3g; Fiber: 1g;
Net carbs: 2g; Protein: 28g;
Macronutrients: Fat: 56%;
Protein: 41%; Carbs: 3%

1. Preheat the oven to 350°F. Line a baking sheet with parchment paper and spray with cooking spray.
2. In a large bowl, mix together the chicken, egg, flour, salt, onion powder, and pepper until well combined.
3. In a medium bowl, combine the pork rinds, parmesan, oregano, garlic powder, and paprika.
4. Scoop the chicken mixture 1 tablespoon at a time and form into your chosen shape. Completely coat in the pork and parmesan mixture and place on the prepared baking sheet.
5. Bake for 15 minutes, flip, and bake for an additional 15 minutes until golden.
6. Serve immediately, refrigerate for up to 5 days, or freeze for up to 3 months. To reheat from frozen, cook at 425°F for 5½ minutes per side.

Chicken Parmesan

SERVES 4 | PREP TIME: 20 MINUTES | COOK TIME: 25 MINUTES

Although the traditional dish is battered in egg and bread crumbs before being deep-fried, this recipe omits the egg and subs out the bread crumbs. Plus, it is sautéed to stay crisp without the hassle of deep-frying. Serve this chicken parmesan with a side of Zoodles (page 166) or shirataki noodles or sandwiched between sliced 90-Second Bread (page 158).

2 large boneless chicken breasts (about 1¼ pounds), pounded to ¼ inch thick

½ teaspoon sea salt, divided

¼ cup grated parmesan cheese

¼ cup almond flour

1 tablespoon coconut flour

¾ teaspoon dried basil

¼ teaspoon dried parsley

⅛ teaspoon garlic powder

⅛ teaspoon freshly ground black pepper

2 tablespoons avocado oil, divided

½ cup Marinara Sauce (page 154)

4 tablespoons shredded mozzarella cheese

Per Serving (¼ recipe): Calories: 414; Total fat: 24g; Total carbs: 8g; Fiber: 2g; Net carbs: 6g; Protein: 42g; Macronutrients: Fat: 52%; Protein: 40%; Carbs: 8%

1. Line a baking sheet with parchment paper.
2. Dry the chicken breasts thoroughly and season with the salt; set aside.
3. In a small bowl, combine the parmesan, almond flour, coconut flour, basil, parsley, garlic powder, and pepper. Spread the mixture out on a baking sheet or plate.
4. In a large skillet over medium-high heat, warm 1 tablespoon of oil.
5. Place 1 chicken breast in the parmesan mixture and turn to coat well on both sides. Lay it in the skillet and cook until golden, about 5 minutes per side. Transfer to the prepared baking sheet.
6. Discard the oil from the skillet. Pour in the remaining 1 tablespoon of oil. Coat and cook the second breast.
7. Preheat the oven to broil.
8. Top the chicken breasts with the marinara sauce and mozzarella. Broil for 1 to 2 minutes, until the cheese is browned and bubbly. Serve immediately or refrigerate for up to 4 days.

> **MAKE IT DAIRY-FREE:** Replace the parmesan with finely crushed pork rinds, and either omit the mozzarella or swap it out for almond "cheese" mozzarella-style shreds.

Chicken Cordon Bleu

SERVES 4 | PREP TIME: 20 MINUTES | COOK TIME: 45 MINUTES

What's not to love about chicken cordon bleu? The problem can be that the chicken dries out while the outside crisps. This recipe uses avocado oil mayonnaise and creamy Dijon mustard to lock in the moisture, while the crushed pork rinds add an extra layer of juicy, fatty richness. You'll need toothpicks to make this recipe.

2 large boneless chicken breasts, pounded to ¼-inch thick
4 slices Swiss cheese
4 slices sugar-free ham
1 teaspoon salt
½ teaspoon freshly ground black pepper
⅓ cup crushed pork rinds
⅓ cup almond flour
¼ cup grated parmesan cheese
1 teaspoon garlic powder
1 teaspoon dried parsley
½ teaspoon paprika
2 tablespoons avocado oil mayonnaise
1 tablespoon Dijon mustard

Per Serving (½ rolled chicken breast): Calories: 417; Total fat: 24g; Total carbs: 6g; Fiber: 1g; Net carbs: 5g; Protein: 46g; Macronutrients: Fat: 52%; Protein: 44%; Carbs: 4%

1. Preheat the oven to 400°F. Line a baking sheet with parchment paper.
2. Dry the chicken breasts thoroughly. Top each with 2 slices of cheese and 2 slices of ham. Roll the breasts up and tuck the ends in to form a tube. Secure with toothpicks and season with the salt and pepper.
3. In a medium bowl, combine the pork rinds, flour, parmesan, garlic powder, parsley, and paprika. Pour the mixture into a shallow dish.
4. In a small bowl, whisk together the mayonnaise and mustard.
5. Brush all sides of each chicken roll with the mayonnaise-mustard mixture; then coat completely with the pork-rind mixture and place on the baking sheet, toothpick-side down.
6. Bake for 30 minutes, rotate the pan, and bake for another 12 minutes until golden.
7. Let sit for 5 minutes before serving. Refrigerate leftovers for up to 4 days. Reheat under a broiler for 3 minutes, watching so the chicken does not burn.

Buffalo Wings

SERVES 4 | PREP TIME: 10 MINUTES | COOK TIME: 45 MINUTES

Crispy wings are often deep-fried before being doused in sauce, but these buffalo wings don't require making a mess. Parboiling the wings draws out some of the fat, helping them crisp up while baking. If spicy wings aren't your thing, replace the hot sauce with ⅓ cup parmesan cheese and 1 teaspoon garlic powder—or simply eat them sauceless. Add a sprinkle of dried parsley before serving, if desired.

2 pounds chicken wings
½ cup (1 stick) salted butter
¾ cup hot sauce

Per Serving (5 wings):
Calories: 637; Total fat: 52g;
Total carbs: 0g; Fiber: 0g;
Net carbs: 0g; Protein: 41g;
Macronutrients: Fat: 73%;
Protein: 27%; Carbs: 0%

1. Preheat the oven to 450°F. Line a baking sheet with paper towels. Line a second baking sheet with parchment paper.
2. Bring a large pot of water to a boil. Add the wings and cook for 6 minutes. Transfer to the baking sheet with paper towels. Cover with another layer of paper towels and pat the wings dry.
3. Place the wings on the second baking sheet in a single layer and bake for 20 minutes per side, 40 minutes total. The skins will be crisp and almost bubbling.
4. While the wings are baking, in a small saucepan over medium heat, melt the butter. Whisk in the hot sauce and reduce the heat to low until ready to use.
5. Remove the wings from the oven and toss them in the hot sauce until evenly coated. Serve immediately or refrigerate for up to 4 days.

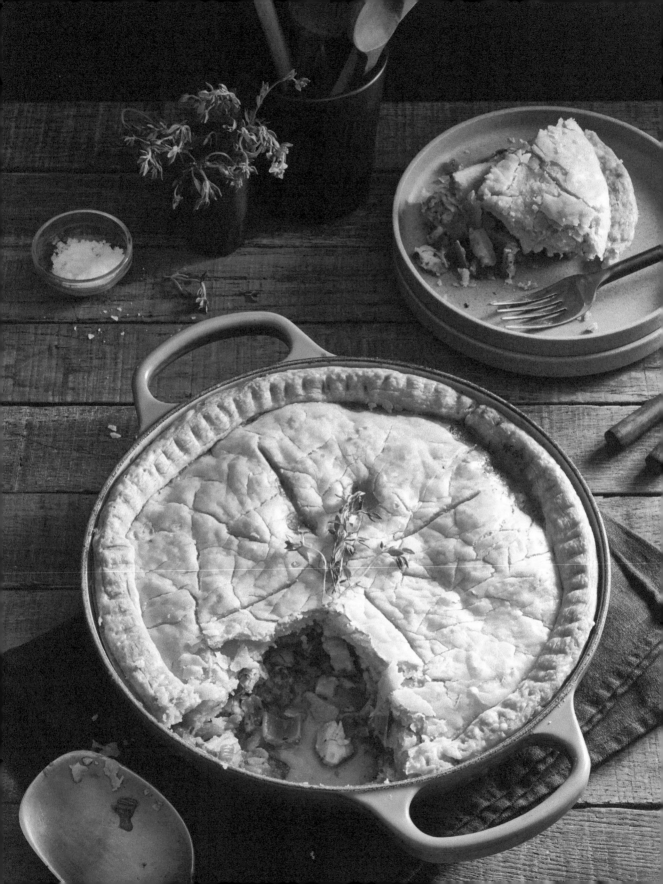

Chicken Pot Pie

SERVES 6 | PREP TIME: 15 MINUTES | COOK TIME: 1 HOUR 5 MINUTES

The flaky, buttery, golden crust of a creamy meat and vegetable pie is what comes to mind when I think of chicken pot pie. My grandmother used to spend an entire day on the crust alone. While a good pot pie takes some time to bake, using fathead dough for the crust saves hours in the kitchen. Consider brushing the top of the dough with a beaten egg for a more golden crust. You can also skip the bottom crust and make this a single-crusted chicken pot pie.

3 tablespoons olive oil
1½ pounds boneless, skinless chicken thighs, cut into 1-inch pieces
¼ cup diced white onion
⅓ cup diced zucchini
⅓ cup diced celery
1 garlic clove, minced
1 teaspoon sea salt
½ teaspoon dried thyme
½ teaspoon dried parsley
1 cup Easy Chicken Bone Broth (page 155) or low-sodium chicken broth
¼ cup heavy cream
¼ teaspoon cream of tartar
Cooking spray
2 recipes Essential Fathead Dough (page 159), formed into 2 balls, chilled
1 egg, beaten (optional)

Per Serving (⅙ recipe): Calories: 639; Total fat: 51g; Total carbs: 10g; Fiber: 3g; Net carbs: 7g; Protein: 39g; Macronutrients: Fat: 72%; Protein: 24%; Carbs: 4%

1. In a large skillet over medium heat, warm the olive oil until shimmering. Add the chicken and cook until browned, about 3 minutes per side.

2. Drop the heat to medium and add the onion, zucchini, and celery. Cook, stirring frequently, until the onions and celery are soft and the zucchini is beginning to brown, about 7 minutes.

3. Stir in the garlic, salt, thyme, and parsley. Cook for 1 more minute.

4. Pour in the broth and scrape the bottom of the pan to release any brown bits. Bring to a boil and then reduce the heat to low and simmer for 20 minutes or until the liquid reduces and the mixture thickens.

5. Slowly pour in the cream and sprinkle in the cream of tartar, whisking constantly. Simmer for another 5 to 10 minutes, until thickened.

6. Preheat the oven to 350°F. Spray a pie dish with cooking spray. Remove the dough from the refrigerator.

CONTINUED ▶

7. Place 1 dough ball at a time between 2 pieces of parchment paper and roll out to ⅛-inch-thick circles.

8. Lay 1 dough circle in the bottom of the pie dish. Pour the pie filling into the dish and then top with the remaining dough circle.

9. Crimp the edges of the dough into the edge of the pie dish. Use a fork to poke holes all over the top of the dough. Brush the dough with the egg (if using), for a darker pie crust.

10. Place the pot pie in the lower third of the oven and bake until the dough is just golden on top, 20 to 25 minutes. Let cool for 5 minutes. Serve immediately or refrigerate for up to 4 days.

Chicken and Dumplings

SERVES 4 | PREP TIME: 15 MINUTES | COOK TIME: 15 MINUTES

Chicken soup may be good for the soul, but adding dumplings takes it to another level of comfort. I was raised on Pennsylvania Dutch chicken and dumplings. Those dumplings were more like thick pieces of egg noodles rather than balls or biscuits, so that's how I make my dumplings now. I love their imperfection: Dumplings should be torn into pieces and look clunky. It's what gives them that comforting charm.

1 tablespoon avocado oil
⅓ cup diced white onion
¼ cup chopped carrots
½ cup chopped celery
2 garlic cloves, minced
1½ cups shredded cooked chicken breast
1 teaspoon dried thyme
4 cups Easy Chicken Bone Broth (page 155)
1 recipe Essential Fathead Dough (page 159)

Per Serving (1¼ cups):
Calories: 454; Total fat: 31g;
Total carbs: 10g; Fiber: 3g;
Net carbs: 7g; Protein: 35g;
Macronutrients: Fat: 61%;
Protein: 31%; Carbs: 8%

1. Heat the avocado oil in a large saucepan over medium heat.
2. Add the onion, carrots, and celery. Cook, stirring frequently, until the onion is translucent, 5 to 6 minutes.
3. Stir in the garlic and cook until fragrant, 1 to 2 minutes. Stir in the chicken and thyme.
4. Pour in the broth and bring to a boil. Reduce the heat to low and simmer while you make the dumplings.
5. Roll the dough into a square ¼ inch thick. Slice the dough into long pieces and then tear into roughly 1-inch chunks.
6. Drop the dumpling pieces into the simmering soup and stir to incorporate.
7. Cook, stirring frequently so the dumplings don't bind together, for another 3 to 5 minutes or until the dumplings are cooked through. Serve immediately.

Chicken Broccoli Rice Casserole

SERVES 6 | PREP TIME: 15 MINUTES | COOK TIME: 30 MINUTES

This dish is a one-pot wonder. It is a creamy, cheesy, low-carb casserole that is simple to make and full of comforting goodness. In this recipe we use the versatile, zero-carb miracle rice in place of white rice, which helps this recipe stay keto-friendly and brings the total cooking time to just 30 minutes. For an extra flavor boost, add ¼ teaspoon each cumin, garlic powder, and paprika to the salt and pepper seasoning.

2 (8-ounce) bags miracle rice, drained and rinsed

1 tablespoon olive oil

¼ cup diced white onion

2 chicken breasts, cut into cubes

2 garlic cloves, minced

¼ teaspoon sea salt

¼ teaspoon freshly ground black pepper

1½ cups low sodium chicken broth

4 ounces full-fat cream cheese, cubed

¼ cup heavy cream

1¼ cups chopped broccoli florets

1 cup shredded cheddar cheese, divided

Salsa, for serving (optional)

Avocado, for serving (optional)

Per Serving (1 cup): Calories: 262; Total fat: 20g; Total carbs: 8g; Fiber: 3g; Net carbs: 5g; Protein: 15g; Macronutrients: Fat: 69%; Protein: 23%; Carbs: 8%

1. Line a baking sheet with paper towels. Spread the rice on the towels and cover with another layer of paper towels. Press down gently to absorb some of the moisture.

2. Heat the oil in a large oven-safe skillet over medium heat. Add the onion and chicken. Cook, stirring frequently, until the chicken browns, 5 to 7 minutes.

3. Stir in the garlic, salt, and pepper until well combined. Cook for 1 more minute. Add the rice and cook until any residual water evaporates, 2 to 3 minutes. Stir in the broth.

4. Drop the heat to low and slowly stir in the cream cheese until completely incorporated. Stir in the cream. Bring the mixture to a boil and then drop the heat to medium low. Cover and cook, stirring occasionally, until the chicken cooks through, about 10 minutes.

5. Stir in the broccoli and ½ cup of cheddar. Cook until the broccoli is tender, 3 to 5 minutes.

6. Preheat the oven to broil.

7. Cover the casserole mixture with the remaining ½ cup of cheddar and broil for 2 minutes, until the cheese bubbles and begins to brown.

8. Let cool slightly before serving. Serve topped with fresh salsa and smashed avocado (if using). Refrigerate for up to 5 days.

Chicken Alfredo

SERVES 4 | PREP TIME: 10 MINUTES | COOK TIME: 30 MINUTES

Juicy chicken thighs swimming in a velvety cheese sauce and served with rich fathead dough noodles make this chicken Alfredo dish one of the most filling keto comfort food dishes I have ever made. As much as I love the versatility and durability of fathead dough noodles, sometimes I crave something lighter. When that craving strikes, I serve this dish over Zoodles (page 166) or freshly steamed garlicky broccoli.

1 recipe Essential Fathead Dough (page 159), rolled into a ball

1 pound boneless skinless chicken thighs, cut into ½-inch slices

1 teaspoon salt

⅛ teaspoon freshly ground black pepper

1 tablespoon olive oil

1 cup chopped broccoli florets

2 tablespoons butter

1 ounce full-fat cream cheese, at room temperature

1 cup heavy cream

⅛ teaspoon nutmeg

¼ teaspoon garlic powder

½ cup shredded parmesan cheese

Per Serving (¼ recipe): Calories: 788; Total fat: 68g; Total carbs: 10g; Fiber: 3g; Net carbs: 7g; Protein: 39g; Macronutrients: Fat: 78%; Protein: 20%; Carbs: 2%

1. Preheat the oven to 400°F.
2. Place the balled dough between 2 pieces of parchment paper. Roll to a ¼-inch thickness.
3. Remove the top paper and place the dough on a baking sheet. Use a fork to poke holes all over. Bake for 12 minutes, until just lightly browned. Cut into fettuccine "noodles" and set aside.
4. Season the chicken with the salt and pepper. In a large skillet over medium heat, warm the oil. Add the chicken and cook, stirring frequently, until it is no longer pink, about 6 minutes. Transfer the chicken to another bowl.
5. In a medium saucepan over high heat, cover the broccoli with water. Cover the pan and bring to a boil. Reduce the heat to medium and cook for 4 to 5 minutes, until the broccoli is fork-tender. Drain completely and set aside.
6. While the broccoli steams, melt the butter in the skillet over medium-high heat. Reduce the heat to medium low after the butter melts, and stir in the cream cheese until melted.

7. Slowly pour in the cream and then sprinkle in the nutmeg and garlic powder. Whisk until thoroughly combined. Bring to a boil and then reduce the heat to simmer and cook until the cream reduces and thickens. Remove from the heat.

8. Stir in the parmesan, chicken, and broccoli. Finally, add the noodles and toss to combine. Serve, or refrigerate for up to 2 days.

LOVING YOUR LEFTOVERS: The butter will separate from the sauce if reheated on too high a heat. Slowly reheat the mixture in a skillet over medium-low heat.

Chicken Fajitas

SERVES 4 | PREP TIME: 15 MINUTES | COOK TIME: 25 MINUTES

Chicken fajitas are a quick, comforting meal that can be made on one baking sheet. Serve them wrapped in lettuce or with a side of tortillas for fellow diners who are not keto. Create your own fixin's bar with fresh salsa, sliced avocado, sour cream, shredded cheese, hot sauce, and lime wedges.

1½ pounds boneless skinless chicken thighs, cut into 1-inch pieces

1 small green bell pepper, cut into strips

1 small red bell pepper, cut into strips

1 small white onion, halved and sliced

1 teaspoon sea salt

1 teaspoon ground cumin

¾ teaspoon paprika

¾ teaspoon chili powder

¾ teaspoon dried oregano

½ teaspoon garlic powder

¼ teaspoon freshly ground black pepper

3 tablespoons avocado oil

Per Serving (¼ recipe): Calories: 312; Total fat: 21g; Total carbs: 5g; Fiber: 1g; Net carbs: 4g; Protein: 28g; Macronutrients: Fat: 60%; Protein: 36%; Carbs: 4%

1. Preheat the oven to 400°F. Line a baking sheet with parchment paper.
2. In a large bowl, combine the chicken, bell peppers, and onion.
3. In a small bowl, combine the salt, cumin, paprika, chili powder, oregano, garlic powder, and pepper.
4. Pour the seasoning mix into the chicken and vegetables and stir well to combine.
5. Add the avocado oil and stir to coat the chicken and vegetables thoroughly.
6. Spread the mixture in a single layer on the prepared baking sheet.
7. Bake for 23 minutes or until the veggies are tender and the chicken is cooked through. Serve immediately or refrigerate for up to 4 days.

Turkey Bacon Ranch Casserole

SERVES 6 | PREP TIME: 15 MINUTES | COOK TIME: 25 MINUTES

If we have leftover turkey, this is my go-to casserole that feeds my entire family. I always look for brands of ranch dressing that use avocado oil instead of corn, vegetable, soy, or other hydrogenated oils. Sir Kensington's and Primal Kitchen are my go-to brands.

1 tablespoon butter
1 pound ground turkey
¾ teaspoon sea salt
¼ teaspoon freshly ground black pepper
4 slices bacon, cooked and chopped
10 ounces frozen spinach, thawed and thoroughly drained
1 garlic clove, minced
½ cup ranch dressing
½ cup shredded mozzarella cheese, divided
½ cup shredded cheddar cheese, divided

Per Serving (⅙ recipe): Calories: 400; Total fat: 32g; Total carbs: 3g; Fiber: 1g; Net carbs: 2g; Protein: 27g; Macronutrients: Fat: 72%; Protein: 27%; Carbs: 1%

1. Preheat the oven to 375°F.
2. In a large skillet over medium heat, melt the butter. Add the turkey and season with the salt and pepper. Cook, breaking up the turkey with a spoon, until it is browned. Set aside.
3. In a large bowl, combine the turkey, bacon, spinach, garlic, ranch dressing, ¼ cup of mozzarella, and ¼ cup of cheddar. Pour into an 8-by-8-inch casserole dish.
4. Top the mixture with the remaining cheeses and bake for 15 to 18 minutes, until the cheese is bubbling and slightly browned. Serve immediately or refrigerate for up to 4 days.

LOVING YOUR LEFTOVERS: When you have leftover Whole Roasted Chicken (page 92), you can use it to make this tasty casserole.

Turkey Tetrazzini

SERVES 4 | PREP TIME: 25 MINUTES | COOK TIME: 30 MINUTES

As a busy mom, I love that this recipe comes together in just 30 minutes and requires only one skillet. To go dairy-free, I use cashew milk in place of the cream, add 2 ounces of almond cream "cheese," and use almond mozzarella shreds instead of cow's milk mozzarella.

1 tablespoon avocado oil
¼ cup diced white onion
1 cup sliced mushrooms
1 garlic clove, minced
2 cups chopped
   cooked turkey
1 teaspoon sea salt
½ teaspoon dried basil
½ teaspoon dried parsley
¼ teaspoon freshly ground
   black pepper
¾ cup heavy cream
¼ teaspoon cream of tartar
1 cup Zoodles (page 166)
½ cup shredded
   mozzarella cheese

Per Serving (1 heaping cup):
Calories: 326; Total fat: 25g;
Total carbs: 6g; Fiber: 1g;
Net carbs: 5g; Protein: 21g;
Macronutrients: Fat: 69%;
Protein: 26%; Carbs: 5%

1. Preheat the oven to 400°F.
2. Heat the oil in a large oven-safe skillet over medium heat. Add the onion and mushrooms and cook until the onions are translucent and the mushrooms begin to brown, 5 to 6 minutes.
3. Stir in the garlic and cook for 1 more minute. Add the turkey and season everything with the salt, basil, parsley, and pepper.
4. Reduce the heat to medium-low and slowly stir in the cream. Bring to a boil and then reduce the heat to a simmer for 2 minutes.
5. Remove from the heat and whisk in the cream of tartar until thoroughly combined. Return the skillet to low heat.
6. Squeeze any remaining water from the zoodles and stir into the turkey mixture until completely combined. Spread the mozzarella cheese evenly on top.
7. Bake for 15 to 20 minutes, until the cheese browns and bubbles. Serve immediately or refrigerate for up to 4 days.

> **SUBSTITUTION TIP:** This dish works just as well with an equal amount of chicken breast rather than turkey.

Turkey Burgers

SERVES 4 | PREP TIME: 10 MINUTES | COOK TIME: 10 MINUTES

Move over beef, it's turkey time! Ground turkey tends to be very lean, meaning it can dry out while cooking. This recipe's avocado adds richness of flavor and protects the meat from drying out. Customize this recipe by topping the burgers with cheese, bacon, tomatoes, onions, and/or your favorite low-carb condiments.

20 ounces ground turkey
1 teaspoon salt
¾ teaspoon paprika
¾ teaspoon ground cumin
½ teaspoon dried oregano
¼ teaspoon garlic powder
⅛ teaspoon freshly ground
    black pepper
2 tablespoons
    almond flour
1 large egg, beaten
1 large Hass avocado, cut
    into cubes
1 tablespoon avocado oil
4 large lettuce leaves

Per Serving (1 burger):
Calories: 522; Total fat: 39g;
Total carbs: 6g; Fiber: 4g;
Net carbs: 2g; Protein: 39g;
Macronutrients: Fat: 67%;
Protein: 30%; Carbs: 3%

1. In a large bowl, combine the turkey, salt, paprika, cumin, oregano, garlic powder, pepper, flour, and egg. Mix until thoroughly combined.

2. Gently fold the avocado chunks into the mixture.

3. Form the mixture into 4 equal patties no more than ½ inch thick.

4. Heat the oil in a skillet over medium-high heat. Cook the burgers for 5 minutes per side, or until they are browned and crisped and the middle of each burger feels firm (not rock solid) to the touch.

5. Serve each burger wrapped inside a large lettuce leaf, or refrigerate for up to 3 days. The avocado may brown a bit, but that is natural.

PREPARATION TIP: Turkey burgers can also be grilled. Turn the grill heat to medium high and spray it with cooking oil. Cook for 5 minutes per side. The burgers are cooked when you place your thumb in the middle of the burger, and it feels firm.

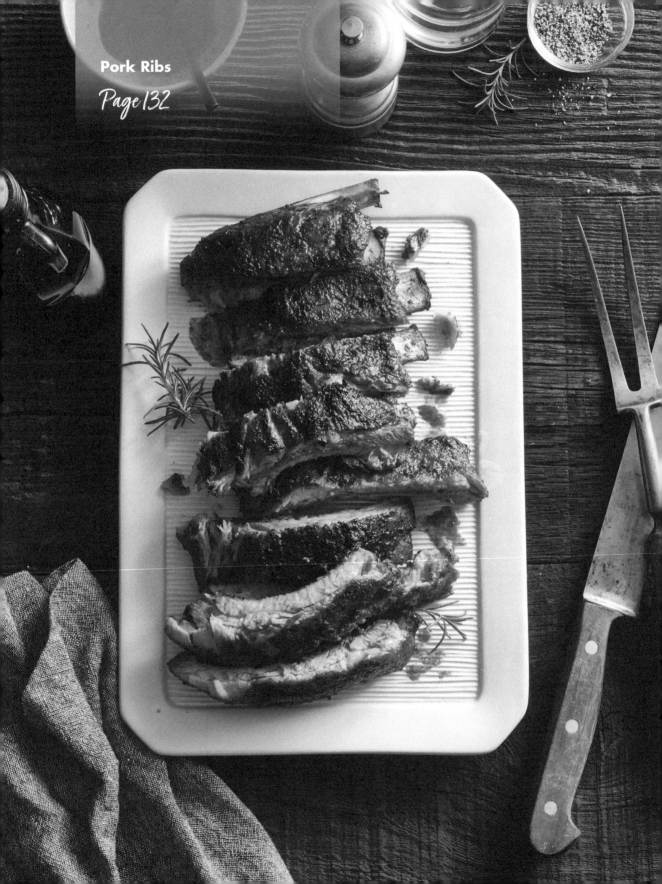

Pork Ribs

Page 132

Chapter 7

BEEF AND PORK

Classic Meatloaf

Meatloaf reminds me of my favorite Christmas movie. Fortunately for me, I have not had to bribe any of my kids to act like a piggy in order to devour this classic meatloaf; they happily scarf it down on their own terms. I find that meatloaf cooks faster when it sits on a baking sheet rather than in a loaf pan. One note: Thoroughly combine the ingredients, but be gentle when mixing to avoid a tough loaf.

⅓ cup tomato sauce
2 tablespoons brown
   sugar alternative
1 tablespoon avocado oil
1 teaspoon Dijon mustard
1 tablespoon olive oil
⅓ cup chopped
   white onion
1 garlic clove, minced
20 ounces ground beef
1 teaspoon sea salt
1 teaspoon dried parsley
¼ teaspoon freshly ground
   black pepper
1 large egg, beaten
2 tablespoons
   melted butter
2 teaspoons
   Worcestershire sauce
¾ cup crushed pork rinds
¼ cup grated
   parmesan cheese

Per Serving (1 slice): Calories: 376; Total fat: 27g; Total carbs: 7g; Fiber: <1g; Net carbs: 6g; Protein: 29g; Macronutrients: Fat: 65%; Protein: 31%; Carbs: 4%

1. Preheat the oven to 350°F. Line a baking sheet with parchment paper.
2. In a small bowl, whisk together the tomato sauce, brown sugar alternative, avocado oil, and mustard. Set aside.
3. Heat the olive oil in a large skillet over medium heat. Add the onion and cook until translucent, 3 to 5 minutes. Stir in the garlic and cook for 1 more minute. Set aside.
4. In a large bowl, combine the beef, salt, parsley, pepper, egg, butter, Worcestershire, and cooked onion and garlic. Using your hands, gently mix everything together by grabbing the meat's outer edge and folding it into the middle, repeating this process until everything is incorporated.
5. Add the pork rinds and parmesan and gently combine.
6. Transfer the mixture to the prepared baking sheet. Shape it into a loaf and slightly flatten the top.
7. Bake for 40 minutes, remove from the oven, and spoon the tomato sauce mixture on top. Bake for an additional 20 to 25 minutes.
8. Let cool for 5 minutes before serving. Refrigerate leftovers for up to 5 days.

Salisbury Steak

SERVES 4 | PREP TIME: 15 MINUTES | COOK TIME: 35 MINUTES

Salisbury steak is basically just a hamburger, but one covered and cooked in thick, rich gravy. Select the fattiest ground beef you can find, preferably at least 80/20, to lock in the juicy texture and add flavor to the mushroom onion sauce. Serve over Buttery Caulimash for a complete comfort food meal.

1 pound 80/20 ground beef
1 teaspoon sea salt, divided
½ teaspoon freshly ground
   black pepper, divided
1 garlic clove, minced
1 large egg, beaten
¼ cup crushed pork rinds
1 tablespoon butter
2 tablespoons olive oil
¼ cup diced white onion
1½ cups sliced mushrooms
2 cups beef broth
2 teaspoons
   Worcestershire sauce
½ teaspoon garlic powder
½ teaspoon
   dried rosemary
¼ cup full-fat sour cream,
   at room temperature
1 recipe Buttery Caulimash
   (page 58)

Per Serving (¼ recipe):
Calories: 637; Total fat: 51g;
Total carbs: 8g; Fiber: 3g;
Net carbs: 5g; Protein: 37g;
Macronutrients: Fat: 72%;
Protein: 23%; Carbs: 5%

1. In a large bowl, combine the beef, ½ teaspoon of salt, ¼ teaspoon of pepper, garlic, egg, and pork rinds. Use your hands to gently mix the ingredients together until well combined. Form into 4 equal-size patties and set aside.

2. Melt the butter in a large skillet over medium-high heat. Cook the patties for 4 minutes per side, until browned and slightly crisped. Set aside.

3. In the same skillet over medium heat, heat the olive oil. Add the onion and mushrooms and cook, stirring frequently, until the onions are translucent and the mushrooms begin to brown, 5 to 6 minutes.

4. Stir in the broth, Worcestershire sauce, remaining ½ teaspoon of salt and ¼ teaspoon of pepper, garlic powder, and rosemary, scraping any brown bits off the bottom of the skillet.

5. Bring the sauce to a boil and then reduce the heat to medium-low to simmer for 5 minutes. Remove from the heat and whisk in the sour cream until thoroughly combined.

6. Return the skillet to medium-low heat. Add the meat patties, cover, and simmer for 10 minutes.

7. Serve over the caulimash. Refrigerate for up to 3 days.

Beef Pot Roast

SERVES 6 | PREP TIME: 15 MINUTES | COOK TIME: 5 HOURS

The secret to a good pot roast is tender, flavorful meat and a rich, hearty gravy. For the beef to achieve that melt-in-your-mouth fork tenderness, it must be seared on each side to lock in the juices and then quickly cooked at a high heat before slow roasting to perfection. You'll get the added benefit of a deliciously aromatic home.

3 tablespoons olive oil, divided

½ tablespoon sea salt, plus 2 teaspoons, divided

1 teaspoon dried thyme

1 teaspoon onion powder

½ teaspoon freshly ground black pepper

3 pounds beef chuck roast, fat untrimmed

½ small white onion, quartered

2 celery stalks, quartered

1 cup quartered radishes

1 cup large cauliflower florets

3 cups beef broth

1 tablespoon Worcestershire sauce

3 garlic cloves, minced

¼ cup heavy cream

1 tablespoon Dijon mustard

¼ teaspoon cream of tartar

Per Serving (⅙ recipe): Calories: 663; Total fat: 50g; Total carbs: 4g; Fiber: 1g; Net carbs: 3g; Protein: 46g; Macronutrients: Fat: 68%; Protein: 28%; Carbs: 4%

1. Preheat the oven to 425°F. Place a skillet over high heat.

2. In a small bowl, combine 2 tablespoons of oil, ½ tablespoon of salt, thyme, onion powder, and pepper. Coat the roast all over with the mixture.

3. Place the roast in the hot skillet and sear until lightly browned on all sides, about 4 minutes per side. Set aside.

4. In a roasting dish, toss the onion, celery, radishes, and cauliflower with the remaining 2 teaspoons of salt and 1 tablespoon of oil. Place the roast directly on top of the vegetables.

5. In another bowl, whisk together the broth, Worcestershire, and garlic. Pour the mixture over the meat and vegetables.

6. Cover the roasting dish with enough aluminum foil so none of the meat or vegetables are visible. Roast for 30 minutes.

7. Remove the roast and reduce the heat to 300°F. Keep it covered in foil. When the temperature is 300°F, return the roast to the oven and cook for 4 hours. The meat is done when it is tender enough to be shredded with a fork.

8. Let the roast sit at room temperature while you prepare the gravy.

9. Ladle 2 cups of cooking liquid into a large saucepan over medium-high heat. Whisk in the cream and then the mustard. Sprinkle in the cream of tartar and whisk vigorously until completely combined.

10. Bring to a boil; then reduce the heat to medium low and simmer for 6 to 7 minutes or until reduced and thickened.

11. To serve, transfer the roast and vegetables to a large platter and slice the meat. Pour the gravy directly on top of the meat and vegetables. Refrigerate the meat and vegetables separately from the gravy for up to 5 days.

PREPARATION TIP: Keep the fat on the roast. It adds more flavor and tenderness and prevents the beef from drying out as it slow roasts.

Beef Stroganoff

SERVES 4 | PREP TIME: 15 MINUTES | COOK TIME: 25 MINUTES

Although zoodles make an excellent keto-friendly swap for noodles, a sturdier substitution is needed to envelope chunks of tender sirloin in a creamy mushroom gravy. Pillowy-soft egg noodles cling to the beef, onions, mushrooms, and spices in this recipe, which is a perfect comfort food dish.

FOR THE EGG NOODLES

Cooking spray
2 ounces full-fat cream cheese, at room temperature
2 tablespoons butter, at room temperature
4 tablespoons almond flour
3 large eggs
¼ teaspoon sea salt

FOR THE BEEF

1 tablespoon olive oil
1 pound sirloin steak tips
1½ teaspoons salt, divided
¼ teaspoon freshly ground black pepper, divided
1 tablespoon butter
¼ cup diced white onion
1¼ cups sliced mushrooms
¼ teaspoon garlic powder
½ cup beef broth
¼ cup heavy cream
⅛ teaspoon nutmeg
¼ teaspoon cream of tartar
½ cup sour cream

Per Serving (1¼ cups): Calories: 606; Total fat: 46g; Total carbs: 7g; Fiber: 1g; Net carbs: 6g; Protein: 44g; Macronutrients: Fat: 68%; Protein: 29%; Carbs: 3%

TO MAKE THE EGG NOODLES

1. Preheat the oven to 300°F. Line a baking sheet with parchment paper and spray the paper with cooking spray.
2. Combine the cream cheese, butter, flour, eggs, and salt in a blender or food processor and blend until smooth.
3. Pour the mixture onto the prepared baking sheet and use a spatula to spread it evenly.
4. Bake for 8 minutes, until lightly browned and no longer jiggly. Let sit at room temperature until cool enough to handle.
5. For even noodles, roll the cooked dough from one end of the baking sheet to the other, forming a tube. Slice horizontally into ¼-inch-thick slices. Unravel the egg noodles and set aside.

TO MAKE THE BEEF

6. In a large skillet over medium-high heat, heat the oil. Stir in the beef and season with 1 teaspoon of salt and ⅛ teaspoon of pepper.
7. Cook, stirring occasionally, for 4 minutes or until the meat is just cooked through. Transfer to a bowl and set aside.

8. Leaving the beef juices in the skillet, melt the butter over medium heat. Add the onions, mushrooms, remaining ½ teaspoon of salt, remaining ⅛ teaspoon of pepper, and the garlic powder. Sauté for 5 to 6 minutes, stirring occasionally, until the onions are translucent. Transfer to the bowl with the beef.

9. In the same skillet over medium-low heat, combine the broth, cream, and nutmeg. Whisk until well combined, scraping the skillet to get the beef and vegetable bits incorporated into the sauce.

10. Whisk in the cream of tartar until completely combined. Allow the sauce to bubble and thicken for 3 to 4 minutes. Reduce the heat to low and whisk in the sour cream until thoroughly combined and the sauce becomes smooth.

11. Return the beef and vegetables to the skillet. Add the egg noodles and stir together until completely combined. Serve immediately or refrigerate for up to 2 days.

SUBSTITUTION TIP: Ground beef can be used instead of sirloin tips. Instead of olive oil, brown the beef in 1 tablespoon of butter. Follow the remaining steps.

Beef and Broccoli Stir-Fry

SERVES 4 | PREP TIME: 15 MINUTES | COOK TIME: 25 MINUTES

Beef and broccoli used to be my go-to when ordering Chinese takeout. The thick brown sauce is loaded with MSG, which is probably what made it taste so good! Many recipes for beef and broccoli brown sauce include hard-to-find ingredients and carb-heavy cornstarch. This one, though, uses coconut aminos, which is thicker than soy sauce and found at most grocery stores. You can use soy sauce, but the sauce will not be as thick or gluten free.

1 tablespoon coconut oil
1 cup Caulirice (page 163)
1 teaspoon sea salt, divided
1 scallion, chopped
1 pound flank steak, cut into thin strips
¼ teaspoon freshly ground black pepper
2 tablespoons avocado oil, divided
2 cups chopped broccoli florets
½ cup water
½ tablespoon coconut aminos
2 teaspoons granular erythritol
1 garlic clove, minced
1 teaspoon ground ginger

Per Serving (¼ recipe): Calories: 351; Total fat: 21g; Total carbs: 8g; Fiber: 2g; Net carbs: 6g; Protein: 37g; Macronutrients: Fat: 54%; Protein: 42%; Carbs: 4%

1. Melt the coconut oil in a large skillet over medium-high heat. When hot, add the cauli-rice and season with ½ teaspoon of salt. Cook, stirring frequently, for 4 minutes. Stir in the scallion and cook for 1 more minute. Transfer to a bowl and set aside.

2. Season the flank steak with the remaining ½ teaspoon of salt and the pepper.

3. Heat 1 tablespoon of avocado oil in the skillet over medium heat. Add the steak and cook, stirring frequently, for 5 to 6 minutes or until the meat is cooked through. Transfer to a bowl and set aside.

4. In the same skillet, heat the remaining 1 tablespoon of avocado oil. Add the broccoli and cook until fork-tender, 6 to 7 minutes, stirring frequently.

5. In a bowl, whisk together the water, coconut aminos, erythritol, garlic, and ginger.

6. Return the beef to the skillet and pour in the coconut aminos mixture. Simmer for 4 to 5 minutes.

7. Serve the stir-fry over the caulirice or refrigerate together for up to 4 days.

> **SUBSTITUTION TIP:** Any protein can be used in place of the flank steak, including sliced chicken breast, boneless pork chops, and large shrimp. Cooking time will vary depending on the protein type. Be sure that each protein is cooked through before moving to step 4.

Spaghetti and Meatballs

SERVES 4 | PREP TIME: 20 MINUTES | COOK TIME: 20 MINUTES

Years ago at an Italian market in Philadelphia, I was buying ground beef to make meatballs. The butcher stopped me from making an all-beef purchase and explained that the best flavor comes from a combination of beef, pork, and veal. It is possible to make this recipe with just beef, but once you taste meatballs made with this medley, you'll be totally sold on the butcher's advice.

1 pound ground beef
½ pound ground pork
½ pound ground veal
1 teaspoon sea salt
1 teaspoon Italian seasoning
¼ teaspoon freshly ground black pepper
1 garlic clove, minced
1 tablespoon melted butter
2 tablespoons grated parmesan cheese
½ cup almond flour
1 large egg, beaten
1 recipe Zoodles (page 166)
2 cups Marinara Sauce (page 154)

Per Serving (¼ recipe):
Calories: 826; Total fat: 57g;
Total carbs: 16g; Fiber: 5g;
Net carbs: 11g; Protein: 63g;
Macronutrients: Fat: 62%;
Protein: 31%; Carbs: 7%

1. Preheat the oven to 400°F. Line a baking sheet with aluminum foil.
2. Combine the beef, pork, veal, salt, Italian seasoning, pepper, garlic, butter, parmesan, flour, and egg in a large bowl. Using your hands, gently combine the ingredients. It's important that you are light with your touch to keep these meatballs nice and juicy.
3. Roll the mixture into 20 equal-size balls and place on the prepared baking sheet. Bake for 20 minutes or until cooked through.
4. While the meatballs bake, in a large pan over low heat, cook the zoodles, stirring, for 1 to 2 minutes. If any water is released during the cooking, simply drain it into the sink.
5. Pour the marinara sauce into the pan and stir until the zoodles are coated in sauce.

6. When the meatballs are ready, add them to the pan with the sauce and zoodles and gently stir to combine. Serve immediately or refrigerate for up to 4 days.

SUBSTITUTION TIP: Shirataki noodles can replace the zoodles to reduce the total carbs. Rinse them thoroughly and then lightly press them between paper towels. Remove the top layer of paper towels and air-dry the noodles for 15 to 20 minutes before cooking.

Beef Stew

SERVES 6 | PREP TIME: 10 MINUTES | COOK TIME: 2 HOURS 25 MINUTES

Hearty, filling, thick, and comforting, this beef stew is all I want to eat when it's cold outside. Instead of using flour or cornstarch to thicken the beef stew, this recipe uses the stew mixture itself. Genius, right? This method can be used in other soup and stew recipes, too. Try it here first so you get the hang of it; then anytime you want a thicker, creamier bowl of soup without adding starch, you'll know what to do.

1 tablespoon olive oil
2 pounds beef stew meat
1½ teaspoons sea salt, divided
¼ teaspoon freshly ground black pepper
⅓ cup diced white onion
1 cup sliced celery
1 garlic clove, minced
1 teaspoon dried thyme
4 cups beef broth
1 bay leaf
1½ cups chopped cauliflower florets
1 cup sliced zucchini

Per Serving (1 cup): Calories: 549; Total fat: 42g; Total carbs: 4g; Fiber: 1g; Net carbs: 3g; Protein: 38g; Macronutrients: Fat: 69%; Protein: 28%; Carbs: 3%

1. Heat the oil in a large stockpot over medium-high heat. Season the beef with 1 teaspoon of salt and the pepper.

2. Add half the meat to the pot and brown on all sides. Transfer to a bowl. Repeat with the remaining meat. Set aside.

3. Keeping the beef fat in the pot, stir in the onion and celery. Cook for 5 to 6 minutes until the onion is translucent. Stir in the garlic, remaining ½ teaspoon of salt, and the thyme and cook for 1 more minute.

4. Add the beef, broth, and bay leaf. Scrape the bottom of the pot to loosen the browned bits.

5. Bring the mixture to a boil and then reduce the heat to low. Cover and cook, stirring occasionally, for 90 minutes or until the beef is tender.

6. Add the cauliflower and zucchini. Stir well to incorporate. Cover and cook, stirring occasionally, for an additional 30 minutes.

7. Remove and discard the bay leaf. Ladle ½ cup of broth with vegetables into a blender. Blend on high until smooth. Return it to the stew and cook for an additional 5 minutes. Serve immediately, refrigerate for up to 5 days, or freeze for up to 3 months.

Oven Burgers

SERVES 4 | PREP TIME: 10 MINUTES | COOK TIME: 25 MINUTES

No grill? No problem. These burgers are cooked to perfection in your oven and ready in about half an hour. Almond butter mixed with ground beef may sound strange, but the creaminess binds the meat and adds to the juicy quality of the burgers. Be sure to use a creamy almond butter, though, or you'll be crunching on almonds while chowing down on your burger.

20 ounces ground beef
1 teaspoon sea salt
1 teaspoon paprika
1 teaspoon garlic powder
¾ teaspoon dried parsley
½ teaspoon freshly ground black pepper
1 large egg, beaten
¼ cup creamy almond butter
8 slices bacon, cooked
½ cup shredded cheddar cheese

Per Serving (1 burger):
Calories: 610; Total fat: 43g;
Total carbs: 5g; Fiber: 2g;
Net carbs: 3g; Protein: 50g;
Macronutrients: Fat: 63%;
Protein: 33%; Carbs: 4%

1. Preheat the oven to 400°F.
2. In a large bowl, combine the beef, salt, paprika, garlic power, parsley, pepper, egg, and almond butter. Gently work the mixture with your hands until the ingredients are thoroughly combined.
3. Press the beef mixture into an 8-by-8-inch baking dish. Bake for 22 minutes. The beef will have shrunken and be swimming in its own juices.
4. Remove from the oven and set the oven to broil.
5. Lay the bacon on top of the oven burger. Top it evenly with the cheddar.
6. Broil for 1 to 2 minutes or until the cheese browns and bubbles.
7. Let cool slightly before cutting into 4 squares and serving. Refrigerate for up to 4 days.

> **SUBSTITUTION TIP:** Oven burgers can be served in large lettuce leaves or sandwiched between sliced 90-Second Bread (page 158) with your favorite toppings.

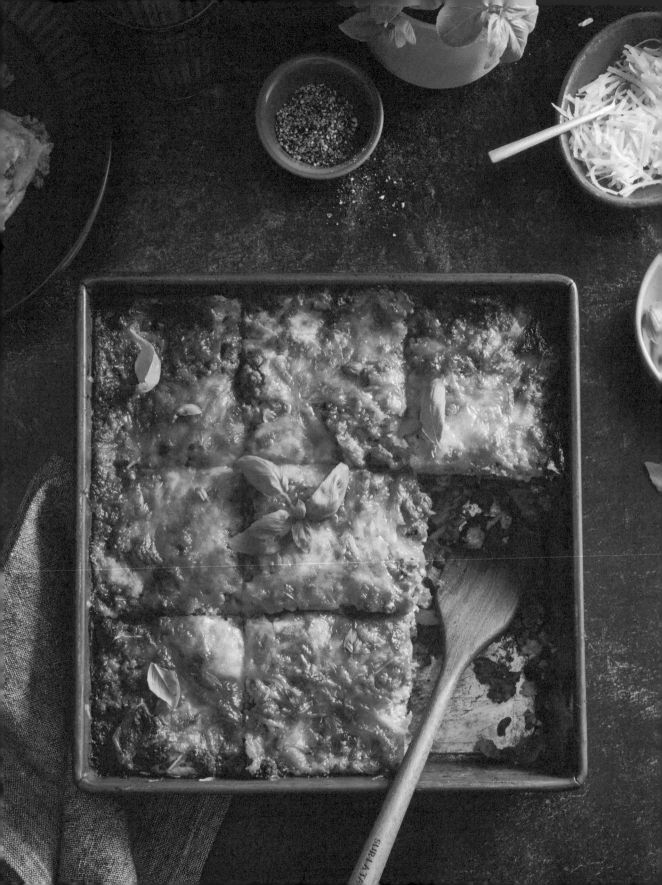

Meat Marinara Lasagna

SERVES 6 | PREP TIME: 20 MINUTES | COOK TIME: 1 HOUR

Making an entire lasagna from scratch—including the noodles and marinara sauce—makes me feel like a professional chef. Using fathead dough to create the noodles is easy and adds another layer of richness to this dish. If you are strapped for time and don't have any homemade marinara, use a sugar-free, low-carb, store-bought brand.

1 recipe Essential Fathead Dough (page 159), rolled into a ball

1½ tablespoons olive oil, divided

1 pound ground beef

½ pound ground Italian sausage

½ small white onion, diced

1 garlic clove, minced

1 recipe Marinara Sauce (page 154)

½ teaspoon sea salt

⅛ teaspoon freshly ground black pepper

1 (8-ounce) container full-fat ricotta cheese, drained, at room temperature, divided

1½ cups shredded mozzarella cheese, divided

½ cup plus 1 tablespoon grated parmesan cheese, divided

Per Serving (⅙ recipe): Calories: 853; Total fat: 65g; Total carbs: 18g; Fiber: 4g; Net carbs: 14g; Protein: 48g; Macronutrients: Fat: 69%; Protein: 23%; Carbs: 8%

1. Preheat the oven to 400°F.

2. Place the balled dough between 2 pieces of parchment paper. Roll into a ¼-inch-thick rectangle.

3. Remove the top paper and place the dough on a baking sheet. Use a fork to poke holes all over. Bake for 12 minutes, until just lightly browned. Cut into six wide lasagna "noodles" and set aside.

4. In a large skillet over medium heat, heat 1 tablespoon of oil. Crumble in the beef and sausage. Brown the meat; then transfer to a bowl and set aside. Discard the fat from the skillet.

5. In the same skillet, heat the remaining ½ tablespoon of oil over medium heat. Add the onion and cook for 3 minutes. Stir in the garlic and cook for 1 more minute. Drop the heat to medium low and stir in the meat and marinara. Season with the salt and pepper.

6. Pour 1 full ladle of meat sauce in the bottom of an 8-by-8-inch baking dish. Lay two lasagna noodles on top. Dollop with one-third of the ricotta, one-third of the meat sauce, ½ cup of mozzarella, and 3 tablespoons of parmesan. Repeat with the remaining ingredients to make 2 more layers.

CONTINUED

7. Bake for about 30 minutes or until the cheese is golden and bubbly. Let sit for 5 minutes before serving. Refrigerate leftovers for up to 5 days.

> **SUBSTITUTION TIP:** Make this recipe with ground chicken or turkey. Add ½ teaspoon sea salt, ¾ teaspoon dried Italian seasoning, and ¼ teaspoon red pepper flakes while browning the poultry in the skillet. Follow the remaining steps.

Sloppy Joes

SERVES 6 | PREP TIME: 15 MINUTES | COOK TIME: 45 MINUTES

Admittedly, I am very type-A in the kitchen and try to avoid making a big mess. When it comes to making sloppy joes, though, the fun is in the mess. When you serve these, make sure to include spoons and forks to get every single bite of the meaty, tomato yumminess.

1 tablespoon butter
1 pound ground beef
1 teaspoon sea salt, divided
¼ teaspoon freshly ground black pepper, divided
1 cup chopped celery
½ small green bell pepper, chopped
½ small red bell pepper, chopped
½ small white onion, chopped
1¼ cups Creamy Tomato Soup (page 45)
1 teaspoon Worcestershire sauce
6 batches 90-Second Bread (page 158), cooled and sliced in half

Per Serving (1 sandwich): Calories: 544; Total fat: 43g; Total carbs: 10g; Fiber: 3g; Net carbs: 7g; Protein: 31g; Macronutrients: Fat: 71%; Protein: 23%; Carbs: 6%

1. Melt the butter in a large skillet over medium heat. Crumble in the beef and season with ½ teaspoon of salt and ⅛ teaspoon of pepper. Cook, stirring frequently and breaking up the meat, until browned and no longer pink. Transfer with a slotted spoon to a bowl and set aside.

2. Reserving the liquid in the skillet, add the celery, bell peppers, and onion. Season with the remaining ½ teaspoon of salt and ⅛ teaspoon of pepper. Cook for 6 to 8 minutes, until softened.

3. Return the beef back to the skillet. Pour in the tomato soup and Worcestershire sauce. Stir well to combine. Bring the mixture to a boil; then reduce the heat to medium low and simmer for 20 minutes or until the meat cooks through and the sauce thickens.

4. Make the 90-Second Bread. When each piece is cool enough to handle, slice in half.

5. Scoop ⅓ cup of sloppy joe onto 6 bread slices. Top with the remaining slices.

6. Serve immediately or refrigerate for up to 5 days or freeze for up to 2 months.

> **SUBSTITUTION TIP:** To keep this recipe even lower in carbs and calories, serve sloppy joes in large lettuce leaves.

Chili con Carne

Chili is a versatile dish that can be served outside of the traditional bowl. Bake it on top of Essential Fathead Dough (page 159) to make a chili pizza. Serve it over a bed of lettuce for a low-carb chili taco salad. Mix it with Zoodles (page 166) or serve it over Caulirice (page 163). You can even use it as a dip for raw vegetable crudités. Switch it up by using ground chicken or turkey instead of beef.

1 tablespoon avocado oil
1 pound ground beef
¼ cup diced white onion
½ small green bell
  pepper, chopped
1 garlic clove, minced
1½ cups canned diced
  tomatoes with liquid
1 cup plain tomato sauce
1 tablespoon chili powder
1 teaspoon sea salt
1 teaspoon ground cumin
½ teaspoon paprika
½ teaspoon freshly
  ground black pepper
1 large Hass
  avocado, sliced

Per Serving (1 cup): Calories: 453; Total fat: 30g; Total carbs: 15g; Fiber: 7g; Net carbs: 8g; Protein: 32g; Macronutrients: Fat: 60%; Protein: 28%; Carbs: 12%

1. Heat the oil in a large stockpot over medium heat. Crumble in the beef.
2. Stir in the onion, bell pepper, and garlic. Cook, stirring frequently, until the beef browns, about 5 minutes.
3. Pour in the tomatoes with their liquid, tomato sauce, chili powder, salt, cumin, paprika, and pepper. Stir to thoroughly combine.
4. Bring the mixture to a boil and then reduce to a simmer over medium-low heat. Cover and cook for 25 minutes until thickened to a stew-like consistency.
5. Serve 1 cup of chili with 2 slices of avocado. Refrigerate leftover chili (without the avocado) for up to 5 days or freeze for up to 3 months.

Pork Chops

SERVES 4 | PREP TIME: 10 MINUTES | COOK TIME: 10 MINUTES

Pork chops and applesauce are an all-American comfort food dish. Instead of actually using applesauce here, we spice the pork chops with apple pie spice. Serve them with a side of Buttery Caulimash (page 58) and Jicama "Apple" Pie Filling (page 151) for a full-on comfort extravaganza.

4 center-cut, bone-in, ¾-inch-thick pork chops
½ teaspoon brown sugar substitute
½ teaspoon ground cinnamon
¼ teaspoon salt
⅛ teaspoon freshly ground black pepper
⅛ teaspoon ground nutmeg
⅛ teaspoon ground ginger
2 tablespoons coconut oil

Per Serving (1 chop): Calories: 252; Total fat: 17g; Total carbs: <1g; Fiber: <1g; Net carbs: <1g; Protein: 23g; Macronutrients: Fat: 61%; Protein: 38%; Carbs: <1%

1. Pat the pork chops dry. Set aside.
2. In a small bowl, combine the brown sugar substitute, cinnamon, salt, pepper, nutmeg, and ginger.
3. Rub both sides of each pork chop with the spice mixture.
4. In a large skillet over medium-high heat, melt the coconut oil.
5. Place the chops in the skillet and cook for 4 to 5 minutes per side, until golden and cooked through. Serve immediately or refrigerate for up to 4 days.

Pork Ribs

SERVES 3 | PREP TIME: 15 MINUTES | COOK TIME: 2 HOURS 5 MINUTES

When baby back ribs are covered with sweet and spice and cooked until they fall off the bone, my taste buds explode. A brown sugar substitute is the secret ingredient to making these pork ribs sweet without adding any sugar; I like Sukrin Gold. It even caramelizes under the broiler while melding into the spices. Add a little more chili powder if you are looking for additional heat.

2 tablespoons avocado oil

1 tablespoon Dijon mustard

2½ tablespoons brown sugar substitute

2 tablespoons paprika

1 tablespoon sea salt

½ tablespoon chili powder

2 teaspoons freshly ground black pepper

3 pounds baby back pork ribs, membranes removed (see tip)

Per Serving (1 pound, about 7 ribs): Calories: 754; Total fat: 43g; Total carbs: 15g; Fiber: 3g; Sugar alcohols: 10g; Net carbs: 2g; Protein: 86g; Macronutrients: Fat: 51%; Protein: 46%; Carbs: 3%

1. Preheat the oven to 300°F. Line a baking sheet with aluminum foil.

2. In a bowl, whisk together the oil, mustard, brown sugar substitute, paprika, salt, chili powder, and pepper.

3. Massage the spice mixture evenly over the front and back of the ribs, covering them completely.

4. Place the ribs on the prepared baking sheet bone-side down. Cover with another layer of foil and bake for 1 hour. Flip the ribs, cover again, and roast for another hour.

5. Remove from the oven and turn the heat to broil. Uncover the ribs and discard the top layer of foil. Flip the ribs back over so the meat side is up. Broil for 4 to 5 minutes, just until the top of the meat begins to crisp.

6. Let the ribs cool slightly before serving. To serve, turn so the ribs are bone-side up and cut between each bone. Refrigerate for up to 4 days. Eat leftovers cold or reheat under a broiler.

> **PREPARATION TIP:** To remove the membrane from the bone side of the ribs, grab one edge of the membrane and slide a butter knife between the membrane and the bone. Hold the loosened membrane with your hands and gently pull it up and back, away from the bones.

Pulled Pork

SERVES 6 | PREP TIME: 15 MINUTES | COOK TIME: 2 HOURS 35 MINUTES

Pulled pork is one of my favorite meals. Pork shoulder—also called pork butt—is an inexpensive cut of meat packed with fatty flavor. Here, we cook this in the oven, but I often throw all the ingredients in the slow cooker and cook on low for 8 to 10 hours overnight. The incredible smell inspires me to get out of bed and start the day.

2 pounds boneless pork shoulder

2 teaspoons sea salt

2 teaspoons freshly ground black pepper

1 tablespoon avocado oil

1 teaspoon ground cumin

1 teaspoon paprika

½ teaspoon dried oregano

2 cups vegetable stock

1 teaspoon orange extract or 1½ tablespoons zest

1 small white onion, sliced

1 bay leaf

Per Serving (4¼ ounces): Calories: 406; Total fat: 31g; Total carbs: 3g; Fiber: 1g; Net carbs: 2g; Protein: 27g; Macronutrients: Fat: 69%; Protein: 27%; Carbs: 4%

1. Cut the pork in half horizontally and then again vertically to get 4 pieces. Season with the salt and pepper.
2. Heat the oil in a large stockpot over high heat. Brown the pork on all sides, about 3 minutes per side, and set aside on a baking sheet. Keep the juices in the pot and remove the pot from the heat.
3. In a small bowl, combine the cumin, paprika, and oregano. Season the pork with the spices. Return the pork to the pot.
4. Pour in the stock and orange extract. Stir in the onion and bay leaf.
5. Bring to a boil and then reduce the heat to medium low. Cover and simmer, stirring occasionally, for 2 hours.
6. Preheat the oven to 450°F.
7. Remove and discard the bay leaf. Transfer the pork, onions, and 1 cup of cooking liquid to a baking dish.
8. Bake for 15 minutes. The pork will be browned on top. Remove from the oven and turn the oven to broil.
9. Shred the pork into the onions and liquid. Return the dish to the oven, broil for 1 minute, stir, and broil for another 2 minutes. Serve immediately or refrigerate in its liquid for up to 5 days.

Pork and Sauerkraut

SERVES 6 | PREP TIME: 10 MINUTES | COOK TIME: 5 HOURS 35 MINUTES

Growing up in Central Pennsylvania, I always ate pork and sauerkraut on New Year's Day. Aside from it being a Pennsylvania Dutch food and family tradition, this dish is eaten on January 1 because it symbolizes good fortune for the coming year. Pork is rich meat (wealth), and sauerkraut is cabbage (money). Making this dish throughout the year is one way to feel healthy, wealthy, and comforted.

¼ cup butter

1 small white onion, sliced

32 ounces sauerkraut in liquid

2 pounds boneless pork shoulder

1½ teaspoons sea salt

¾ teaspoon freshly ground black pepper

1 tablespoon avocado oil

Per Serving (4 ounces pork + 1 cup sauerkraut): Calories: 492; Total fat: 39g; Total carbs: 8g; Fiber: 5g; Net carbs: 3g; Protein: 28g; Macronutrients: Fat: 71%; Protein: 23%; Carbs: 6%

1. Preheat the oven to 250°F.

2. In a large saucepan over medium heat, melt the butter. Add the onion and cook, stirring frequently, until soft and golden.

3. Pour in the sauerkraut and liquid. Stir to thoroughly combine. Drop the heat to medium low and simmer for 15 minutes.

4. While the onions and sauerkraut are simmering, cut the pork into 4 pieces. Season with the salt and pepper.

5. In a large skillet over medium-high heat, brown all sides of the pork. Transfer to a roasting dish. Pour the onion and sauerkraut mixture over the pork. Cover with aluminum foil.

6. Bake for 2 hours and 45 minutes; then rotate the pan and bake for another 2 hours and 30 minutes.

7. Use two forks to shred the pork into the sauerkraut mixture. Serve immediately, refrigerate for up to 5 days, or freeze for up to 3 months.

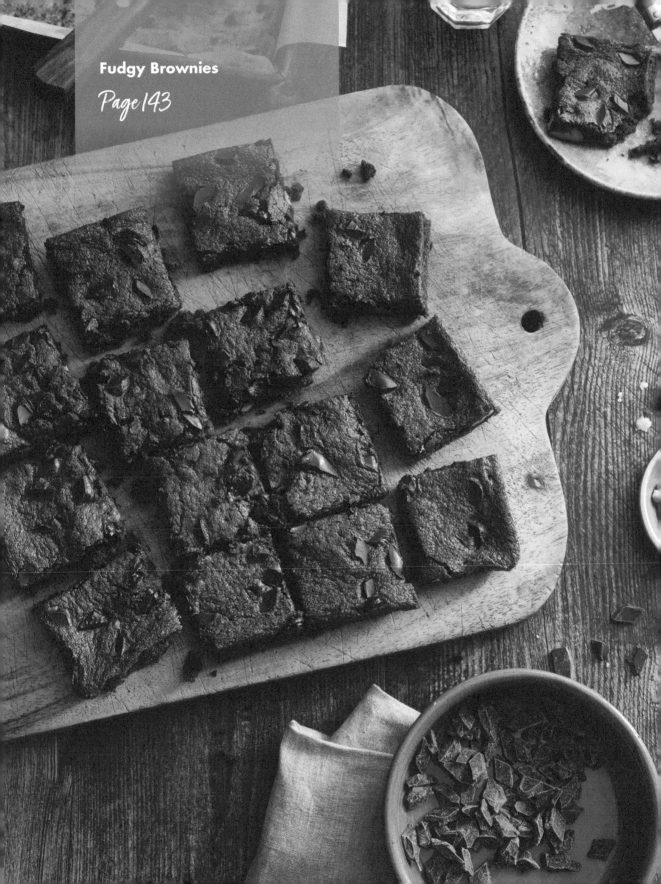

Fudgy Brownies

Page 143

Chapter 8

DESSERTS

Cinnamon Roll Fat Bomb

MAKES 16 | PREP TIME: 15 MINUTES, PLUS 45 MINUTES TO CHILL

During the first six months of my ketogenic journey, I relied on sweet fat bombs to help me conquer my sugar cravings. I'm pretty sure that I avoided going to the mall for those six months because smelling Cinnabon may have thrown me off track. These bombs taste like a bite of cinnamon-bun heaven with the fueling power of fat.

FOR THE BOMBS

¼ cup butter, at room temperature

2 ounces full-fat cream cheese, at room temperature

¼ cup brown sugar replacement

½ cup almond flour

1 teaspoon ground cinnamon

FOR THE ICING

1 tablespoon creamy almond butter

1 tablespoon coconut oil, melted

½ tablespoon powdered erythritol

1 teaspoon ground cinnamon

½ teaspoon vanilla extract

Per Serving (1 bomb): Calories: 72; Total fat: 7g; Total carbs: 5g; Fiber: 1g; Sugar alcohol: 3g; Net carbs: 1g; Protein: 1g; Macronutrients: Fat: 88%; Protein: 6%; Carbs: 6%

TO MAKE THE BOMBS

1. In a large bowl, beat together the butter and cream cheese. Add the brown sugar replacement and beat until well combined. Add the flour and cinnamon and beat until thoroughly blended.

2. Cover the bowl and refrigerate for 15 to 20 minutes, until the dough solidifies.

3. Line a baking sheet with parchment paper. Using a tablespoon, scoop the mixture out of the bowl and use your hands to roll it into balls. Place the balls on the baking sheet.

4. Refrigerate the balls for 1 hour or freeze for 15 minutes, until solid to the touch.

TO MAKE THE ICING

5. While the cinnamon rolls are hardening, make the icing. If the almond butter is not creamy and drippy at room temperature, warm it in the microwave for 20 seconds. If the erythritol is not powdered, whiz it in a blender or food processor for about 30 seconds.

6. In a small bowl, whisk together the almond butter, coconut oil, erythritol, cinnamon, and vanilla.

7. Drizzle the icing mixture evenly over the cold cinnamon balls. Refrigerate or freeze again until the frosting sets. Let sit at room temperature for 5 minutes before serving. Store in an airtight container in the freezer.

> **MAKE IT DAIRY-FREE:** Substitute ghee or coconut oil for the butter and use nut-milk cream cheese. Coconut oil will melt, so it's important to keep these fat bombs as cold as possible, especially if you are making a dairy-free version.

Chocolate Chip Cookies

MAKES 20 | PREP TIME: 15 MINUTES | COOK TIME: 40 MINUTES

These are a staple dessert in my home, served with a big glass of cold unsweetened vanilla almond milk. Browning your butter adds so much richness to these cookies that when I served them to my kids, they insisted I had added sugar.

½ cup (1 stick)
  unsalted butter
1½ cups almond flour
½ teaspoon baking powder
¼ teaspoon cream of tartar
⅛ teaspoon sea salt
½ cup erythritol
¼ cup brown
  sugar replacement
1 large egg, at
  room temperature
1 teaspoon vanilla extract
½ cup sugar-free
  chocolate chips

Per Serving (1 cookie):
Calories: 109; Total fat: 11g;
Total carbs: 12g; Fiber: 2g;
Sugar alcohols: 8g;
Net carbs: 2g; Protein: 2g;
Macronutrients: Fat: 91%;
Protein: 7%; Carbs: 2%

1. In a saucepan over medium-low heat, brown the butter. This will take about 20 minutes, and you need to watch the butter so it browns and doesn't burn. (You will know if the butter has burned if it is smoking and black bits are floating throughout.)

2. Once the butter browns, let cool for 15 minutes.

3. Preheat the oven to 350°F and line a baking sheet with parchment paper.

4. In a large bowl, combine the almond flour, baking powder, cream of tartar, salt, erythritol, and brown sugar replacement.

5. In another large bowl, mix together the egg and vanilla.

6. Using an electric hand mixer or stand mixer, beat half of the dry mix into the eggs and vanilla. Beat in the browned butter and then the remaining dry mix.

7. Stir in the chocolate chips.

8. Scoop tablespoons of dough onto the prepared baking sheet. You should have 20 cookies ready to be baked.

9. Bake for 15 to 17 minutes, until just browned on the edges.

10. Cool at room temperature before removing them from the baking sheet.

11. Enjoy! Store in an airtight container at room temperature for up to 5 days.

PREPARATION TIP: You can kick the healthiness of these cookies up a notch by adding omega-3-rich walnuts. Use ¼ cup sugar-free chocolate chips and ¼ cup walnuts.

Almond Butter Oatmeal Cookies

MAKES 18 TO 20 | PREP TIME: 10 MINUTES, PLUS 20 MINUTES TO CHILL
COOK TIME: 10 MINUTES

I stumbled upon this recipe one day when I mixed together almond butter and sugar-free maple syrup. The taste took me right back to eating those little packets of instant brown sugar and maple oatmeal. I knew I was onto something, and this cookie tastes exactly like a bowl of oatmeal but in a delicious cookie bite.

Butter or cooking spray,
  for greasing (optional)
1 cup unsweetened,
  unsalted almond butter,
  creamy but not liquid
¼ cup sugar-free
  maple-flavored syrup
1 tablespoon brown
  sugar substitute
1¼ teaspoons
  ground cinnamon
½ tablespoon
  baking powder
¼ teaspoon sea salt
1 large egg, beaten

Per Serving (1 cookie): Calories: 93; Total fat: 8g; Total carbs: 4g; Fiber: 2g; Net carbs: 2g; Protein: 3g; Macronutrients: Fat: 77%; Protein: 13%; Carbs: 10%

1. Line 2 nonstick baking sheets with parchment paper or grease them with butter or cooking spray.
2. In a large bowl, beat the almond butter, syrup, brown sugar substitute, cinnamon, baking powder, salt, and egg together until well combined.
3. Scoop tablespoons of dough onto the prepared baking sheets, leaving a solid inch between each cookie because they will spread when baking. Press down gently to form them into cookies.
4. Preheat the oven to 350°F and place the baking sheets in the refrigerator for 20 minutes.
5. Bake the cookies 1 sheet at a time for about 10 minutes, until golden around the edges. Keep the second sheet refrigerated while the other bakes.
6. Cool the cookies completely before removing them from the baking sheet to avoid crumbling. Store in an airtight container at room temperature for up to 5 days. These cookies don't freeze well, so you'll want to gobble them all up or share them.

PREPARATION TIP: If your baking sheets won't fit in the refrigerator, place the unpressed cookie balls in a container, refrigerate, and then press them gently before they go into the oven.

Fudgy Brownies

MAKES 16 | PREP TIME: 15 MINUTES | COOK TIME: 20 MINUTES

There are cakey brownies, and there are fudgy brownies. Give me all the richness of the fudge and save the cakeyness for cake. The key to a fudgy brownie is to not overmix the batter. (That makes them cakey.) These brownies are super fudgy, and when I am feeling extra indulgent, I swap the vanilla for hazelnut to create a Nutella-tasting treat.

5 tablespoons butter, at room temperature
⅔ cup granular erythritol
1 cup almond flour
⅓ cup unsweetened cocoa powder
1 teaspoon baking powder
¼ teaspoon sea salt
2 large eggs at room temperature
1 teaspoon vanilla extract
3 tablespoons unsweetened vanilla almond milk
½ cup sugar-free chocolate chips or chopped walnuts, divided

Per Serving (1 brownie):
Calories: 106; Total fat: 10g;
Total carbs: 14g; Fiber: 3g;
Sugar alcohols: 9g;
Net carbs: 2g; Protein: 3g;
Macronutrients: Fat: 85%;
Protein: 11%; Carbs: 3%

1. Preheat the oven to 350°F. Line an 8-by-8-inch baking dish with parchment paper.

2. In a large bowl, beat together the butter and erythritol until the sweetener dissolves.

3. In another large bowl, whisk together the flour, cocoa powder, baking powder, and salt.

4. Beat half of this dry mixture into the butter; then beat in 1 egg. Repeat with the remaining dry mix and the remaining egg.

5. Beat in the vanilla and then the almond milk. As soon as the almond milk incorporates, stop mixing the batter. It should appear thinner than a cookie batter, resembling a boxed cake mix. Gently fold in half the chocolate chips.

6. Pour the mixture into the prepared dish and top evenly with the remaining chocolate chips.

7. Bake for 20 minutes or until a toothpick inserted in the middle of the dish comes out clean. Don't overbake these; if your oven runs hot, start checking them at 18 minutes.

8. Let the brownies cool at room temperature for at least 30 minutes before slicing and serving. Store in an airtight container or sealed plastic bag for up to 6 days.

Mug Cake Three Ways

MAKES 1 CAKE | PREP TIME: 10 MINUTES | COOK TIME: 1 MINUTE

These recipes use almond milk, flavor extracts, and powders to avoid dry, eggy mug cakes. Be sure to mix the ingredients in a bowl before putting them in the mug. Choose the flavor that best suits you, and if you want icing, use whipped heavy cream or coconut cream.

FOR ALL MUG CAKES
1 tablespoon butter
3 tablespoons almond flour
½ teaspoon baking powder
1 large egg, beaten

FOR A VANILLA MUG CAKE
1½ tablespoons plus 2 teaspoons erythritol
1 tablespoon coconut flour
⅛ teaspoon ground cinnamon
1 tablespoon unsweetened vanilla almond milk
1½ teaspoons vanilla extract
Cooking spray

FOR A CHOCOLATE MUG CAKE
2½ tablespoons unsweetened cocoa powder
1 tablespoon erythritol
1 tablespoon unsweetened vanilla almond milk
Cooking spray

FOR A LEMON MUG CAKE
1½ tablespoons plus 1 teaspoon erythritol
1 tablespoon coconut flour
1 tablespoon unsweetened vanilla almond milk
1 teaspoon lemon zest
1 teaspoon lemon extract
Cooking spray

1. In a small skillet, melt the butter. Let it sit at room temperature for 5 to 10 minutes or until it cools slightly but is still liquid.
2. Pour the cooled butter into a medium-size bowl. Add the almond flour, baking powder, and egg, and whisk until combined.
3. To the same bowl, add all of the ingredients for your chosen mug cake, except the cooking spray, and whisk again.
4. Spray a large microwave-safe mug with cooking spray and pour in the batter.
5. Microwave on high for 60 seconds. If the edges are pulling away from the sides of the mug, but the middle looks slightly underdone, the mug cake is done. If not, cook in 15-second intervals until done.
6. Let the mug cake cool for 1 to 2 minutes. Remove it with a spatula or butter knife or eat it straight out of the mug.

Per Serving (1 vanilla mug cake): Calories: 352; Total fat: 29g; Total carbs: 38g; Fiber: 5g; Sugar alcohols: 28g; Net carbs: 5g; Protein: 12g; Macronutrients: Fat: 74%; Protein: 14%; Carbs: 12%

Per Serving (1 chocolate mug cake): Calories: 334; Total fat: 29g; Total carbs: 25g; Fiber: 7g; Sugar alcohols: 12g; Net carbs: 6g; Protein: 14g; Macronutrients: Fat: 78%; Protein: 17%; Carbs: 5%

Per Serving (1 lemon mug cake): Calories: 334; Total fat: 29g; Total carbs: 34g; Fiber: 5g; Sugar alcohols: 24g; Net carbs: 5g; Protein: 12g; Macronutrients: Fat: 78%; Protein: 14%; Carbs: 8%

Bread Pudding

SERVES 6 | PREP TIME: 10 MINUTES | COOK TIME: 45 MINUTES

You may have been missing bread pudding since going keto, but now you can satisfy the craving. Try different flavor extracts, sprinkle with sugar-free chocolate chips before baking, or serve with a dollop of whipped cream. Or drizzle with sugar-free maple syrup and eat warm for breakfast.

4 batches 90-Second Bread (page 158; see Note)

Cooking spray

¾ cup canned coconut milk

¾ cup unsweetened vanilla almond milk

4 tablespoons melted butter

3 large eggs

¼ cup granular erythritol

1 tablespoon brown sugar substitute

1 teaspoon vanilla extract

½ teaspoon ground cinnamon

Per Serving (⅙ recipe): Calories: 365; Total fat: 34g; Total carbs: 16g; Fiber: 2g; Sugar alcohols: 10g; Net carbs: 4g; Protein: 11g; Macronutrients: Fat: 84%; Protein: 12%; Carbs: 4%

1. Preheat the oven to 375°F. Spray an 8-by-8-inch baking dish with cooking spray.
2. Make the 90-Second Bread. When each piece is cool enough to handle, cut into ½-inch cubes.
3. Add the cubes to the prepared dish and set aside.
4. In a medium saucepan over medium heat, combine the coconut milk and almond milk. Raise the heat to medium high, and just as the mixture begins to bubble, reduce the heat to medium low.
5. Whisk the butter into the milk until thoroughly incorporated. Slowly pour the liquid on top of the bread. Gently stir to ensure each bread cube has been touched by the mixture.
6. In a medium bowl, beat together the eggs, erythritol, and brown sugar substitute. Beat in the vanilla and cinnamon. Keep beating until the eggs look foamy and the sweetener dissolves a bit, about 1 minute.
7. Pour the eggs over the soaked bread cubes.
8. Bake until set, 25 to 30 minutes. It is done when it no longer jiggles.
9. Cool slightly before serving. Refrigerate for up to 2 days. The bread will become mushy, so it is best to reheat in a frying pan.

NOTE: Make the 90-Second Bread using 1 tablespoon coconut oil in lieu of the butter and add ¼ teaspoon cinnamon to the batter.

Rice Pudding

SERVES 3 | PREP TIME: 20 MINUTES, PLUS 2 HOURS TO CHIL | COOK TIME: 20 MINUTES

My husband's favorite dessert of all time is rice pudding. There is only one ingredient I have found that can truly mimic rice (or tapioca for that matter) in a pudding: miracle rice. Like shirataki noodles, miracle rice contains less than 1 gram of carbohydrates for the entire bag. Rinsing and boiling the miracle rice removes the odd smell and neutralizes its flavor, allowing it to fully absorb the rice pudding's flavors.

1 (14.5-ounce) can full-fat coconut milk
1½ tablespoons erythritol
2 cups water
Pinch sea salt
1 (8-ounce) package miracle rice
1 teaspoon vanilla extract
1½ teaspoons ground cinnamon

Per Serving (⅓ recipe):
Calories: 248; Total fat: 24g; Total carbs: 17g; Fiber: 4g; Sugar alcohols: 6g; Net carbs: 7g; Protein: 2g; Macronutrients: Fat: 87%; Protein: 3%; Carbs: 10%

1. Pour the coconut milk into a small saucepan over medium-high heat and bring to a slow boil, whisking occasionally.

2. Once the coconut milk begins to bubble, add the erythritol and whisk until it dissolves. Reduce the heat and simmer, whisking occasionally, for 7 to 10 minutes until the mixture thickens.

3. When it is thick enough to cling to the back of a spoon, pour it into a bowl. Refrigerate for at least 1 hour.

4. Meanwhile, drain and rinse the miracle rice. Bring the water and salt to a boil and add the rice. Boil for 2 minutes; then drain and rinse again under cold water.

5. Add the rice to the thickened coconut milk mixture. Stir in the vanilla and cinnamon.

6. Refrigerate for another hour or overnight before serving. Refrigerate for up to 6 days.

Banana Pudding

MAKES 2 CUPS | PREP TIME: 25 MINUTES, PLUS 2 HOURS TO CHILL | COOK TIME: 10 MINUTES

Every time I visited my godmother, she would make a big bowl of banana pudding just for me. As much as I love the taste of banana, they are too high in sugar to be part of my ketogenic lifestyle, so replicating her dish called for banana extract. Using gelatin instead of eggs creates the pudding texture without the possibility of little cooked egg bits floating in your pudding.

1 (¼-ounce) envelope
   unflavored gelatin
½ cup water
1 cup canned full-fat
   coconut milk or
   heavy cream
½ cup granular erythritol
1 teaspoon banana extract

Per Serving (½ cup): Calories: 108; Total fat: 11g; Total carbs: 27g; Fiber: 1g; Sugar alcohols: 24g; Net carbs: 2g; Protein: 2g; Macronutrients: Fat: 81%; Protein: 8%; Carbs: 11%

1. In a small bowl, whisk together the gelatin and water until the gelatin dissolves. Set aside.

2. Heat the coconut milk in a medium saucepan over medium-low heat. Whisk until the milk is smooth and homogenous.

3. In a blender or food processor, pulse the erythritol a few times until it becomes powdered. (This helps it dissolve better.) Whisk it into the coconut milk and continue to cook, whisking constantly, until the milk thickens and the sweetener dissolves, about 16 minutes.

4. Remove from the heat and very slowly add the gelatin, whisking constantly to ensure no bits of gelatin are present.

5. Return the pan to medium-low heat. Whisk in the banana extract until thoroughly combined.

6. Pour the pudding mixture into a container and cover it with plastic wrap before securing the container's lid. Make sure the plastic wrap touches the surface of the pudding to prevent a hard film from forming. Refrigerate for at least 2 hours, preferably overnight, until set. Serve.

SUBSTITUTION TIP: You can play with different flavored extracts, such as pineapple, and have yourself a piña colada pudding.

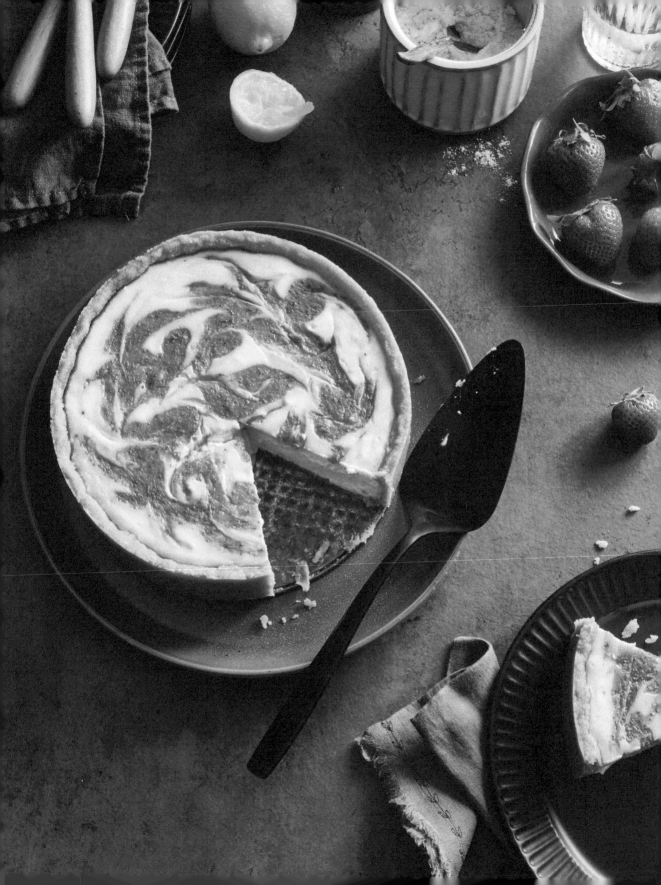

Strawberry Cheesecake

SERVES 12 | PREP TIME: 10 MINUTES, PLUS 9 HOURS 20 MINUTES TO CHILL
COOK TIME: 55 MINUTES

We used to live down the street from a restaurant known for its cheese-cakes. I love to replicate that dish when strawberries are in season because, when picked at their peak, they are plump, juicy, sweet, and flavorful. In fact, I omit the strawberry extract in this recipe when I can buy great strawberries; but for the remainder of the year, the extract really adds an extra punch of strawberry flavor.

1½ cups almond flour

6 tablespoons melted butter

2 tablespoons sugar-free maple syrup

1 tablespoon brown sugar substitute

1 teaspoon ground cinnamon

¾ cup erythritol

1 cup sliced ripe strawberries

2 (8-ounce) packages full-fat cream cheese, at room temperature

1 cup full-fat sour cream, at room temperature

¾ teaspoon vanilla extract

¾ teaspoon strawberry extract

½ tablespoon lemon juice

2 large eggs, at room temperature

Per Serving (1 slice): Calories: 322; Total fat: 31g; Total carbs: 21g; Fiber: 2g; Sugar alcohols: 13g; Net carbs: 6g; Protein: 7g; Macronutrients: Fat: 82%; Protein: 8%; Carbs: 10%

1. In a large bowl, combine the almond flour, butter, syrup, brown sugar substitute, and cinnamon. Stir until thoroughly combined; then pour into a 9-inch springform pie pan. Pack it down evenly on the bottom and sides of the pan. Refrigerate for at least 20 minutes until firm to the touch.

2. Preheat the oven to 350°F.

3. Pulse the erythritol in a blender or food processor until powdered. Set aside.

4. Puree the strawberries in a blender. Set aside.

5. In a bowl, gently beat together the cream cheese and sour cream. Add the erythritol, vanilla, strawberry extract, and lemon juice.

6. Beat in one egg at a time until fully incorporated.

7. Pour the cheesecake mixture into the chilled pie crust. Drizzle with the pureed strawberries. Use a butter knife to swirl the puree into the cheesecake.

8. Place the cheesecake dish in a large roasting pan and carefully pour hot water into the pan to reach about halfway up the side of the cheesecake dish. (Hot water adds humidity and prevents the cheesecake from cracking.)

CONTINUED ▶

9. Lay a piece of aluminum foil loosely on top of the roasting pan.

10. Bake for 45 to 55 minutes, until the edges are set, but the center still jiggles. Turn off the oven and crack open the oven door. Leave the cheesecake for 30 minutes.

11. Remove the cheesecake from the water bath. Let sit at room temperature for 1 hour.

12. Cover the cooled cheesecake with plastic wrap and refrigerate for 8 hours or overnight before serving. Refrigerate for up to 1 week or freeze for up to 2 weeks.

Jicama "Apple" Pie Filling

SERVES 4 | PREP TIME: 35 MINUTES | COOK TIME: 1 HOUR

When July 4 rolls around, my taste buds start begging for apple pie. Jicama is a great substitute for apples because it has a relatively neutral flavor and a very similar texture when cooked. Once you peel the jicama root, it even looks like a peeled apple. This recipe's ingredients and cooking method produce a caramel-like apple pie filling. Enjoy it on its own, with a dollop of sugar-free whipped cream, or as filling in a keto-friendly pie crust.

1 tablespoon coconut oil
1½ cups cubed jicama
½ tablespoon ground
   cinnamon
½ teaspoon
   ground nutmeg
¼ teaspoon allspice
2 tablespoons erythritol
1½ teaspoons apple
   extract flavoring
½ cup sugar-free maple
   syrup, divided
1 cup, plus 2 tablespoons
   water, divided

Per Serving (¼ recipe): Calories: 65; Total fat: 4g; Total carbs: 15g; Fiber: 7g; Sugar alcohols: 6g; Net carbs: 2g; Protein: <1g; Macronutrients: Fat: 49%; Protein: <1%; Carbs: 51%

1. In a large saucepan over medium-high heat, melt the coconut oil.
2. Add the jicama and cook, stirring occasionally, for 10 minutes.
3. Add the cinnamon, nutmeg, allspice, erythritol, apple extract, ¼ cup of syrup, and ½ cup plus 1 tablespoon of water. Stir until completely combined.
4. Bring the mixture to a gentle boil; then reduce the heat to medium low and simmer for 25 minutes, stirring occasionally. The mixture will thicken and become sticky, but the jicama will still be crisp.
5. Stir in the remaining ¼ cup of syrup and ½ cup plus 1 tablespoon of water.
6. Continue to simmer, stirring occasionally, for 20 minutes longer or until the jicama is fork-tender.
7. Remove from the heat and let sit for 20 minutes. The sauce will be the texture of a thick but pourable caramel, and the jicama will be tender but still have a crunch.
8. Serve immediately or refrigerate for up to 4 days.

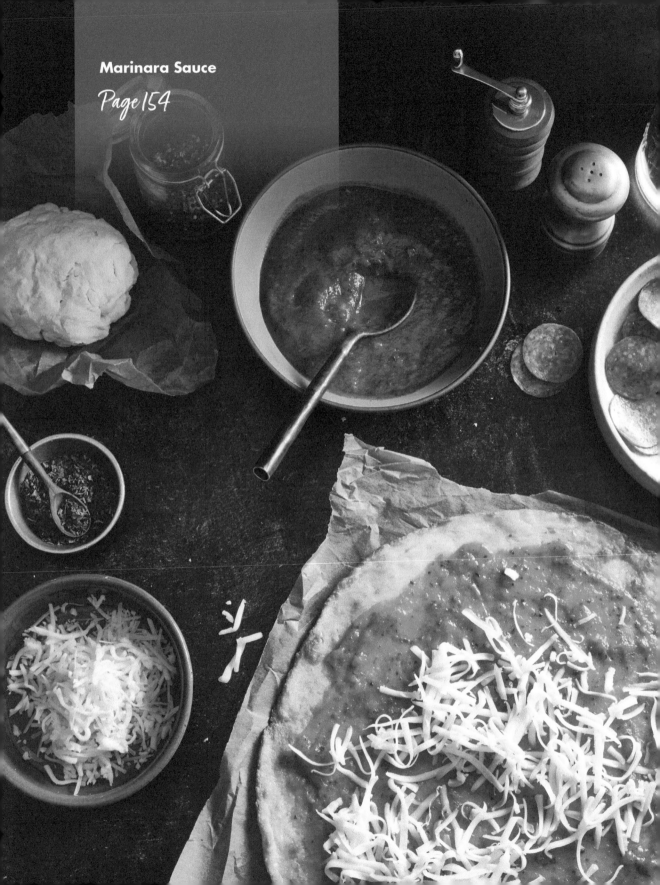

Marinara Sauce

Page 154

Chapter 9

STAPLES, SNACKS, AND DRINKS

Marinara Sauce

MAKES 3 CUPS | PREP TIME: 5 MINUTES | COOK TIME: 30 MINUTES

If you love marinara sauce but find that it gives you heartburn, this recipe is for you. Instead of using onion and garlic for flavor, we substitute celery, carrot, and herbs. These vegetables are lower in acidity and perfect for a sensitive stomach. I like San Marzano tomatoes because they're sweeter and lower in acid than other canned tomato varieties. Grab an apron because cooking this sauce can get a little messy.

1 (28-ounce) can whole plum tomatoes
¼ cup olive oil
2 tablespoons diced carrot
2 tablespoons diced celery
½ teaspoon sea salt
1½ tablespoons dried basil
½ teaspoon garlic powder
½ cup water

Per Serving (½ cup): Calories: 118; Total fat: 9g; Total carbs: 7g; Fiber: 3g' Net carbs: 4g; Protein: 1g; Macronutrients: Fat: 69%; Protein: 3%; Carbs: 28%

1. Pour the entire can of tomatoes into a bowl and crush them with your hands. Set aside.
2. In a large saucepan over medium heat, heat the oil.
3. Stir in the carrots and cook for 4 to 5 minutes, until they begin to soften.
4. Add the celery and salt and cook for another 3 to 4 minutes, stirring to avoid burning.
5. Pour in the tomatoes, basil, garlic powder, and water and stir well.
6. Bring to a boil; then quickly reduce the heat to low and simmer, covered, for 20 minutes.
7. Use an immersion blender or stand blender and blend the sauce completely.
8. Portion into 1-cup serving sizes and either refrigerate for up to 1 week or freeze for up to 3 months.

FEEDING THE FAMILY: Make a Bolognese sauce with ground beef, sausage, chicken, or turkey. Brown the protein in a large skillet over medium heat. Drain excess fat. After blending the marinara sauce, pour it and the protein into a large saucepan. Bring to a boil; then reduce the heat and simmer for 15 to 20 minutes.

Easy Chicken Bone Broth

MAKES 8 CUPS | PREP TIME: 10 MINUTES | COOK TIME: 12 HOURS 30 MINUTES

Save the carcasses of your rotisserie and/or Whole Roasted Chicken (page 92) by storing them in the freezer and pull them out when you are ready to make bone broth. Roasting the bones may seem like an unnecessary step, but it adds a richer flavor to your broth.

2 chicken carcasses
1 tablespoon tomato paste
2 celery stalks, quartered
5 baby carrots
1 small onion, quartered
1 tablespoon apple
   cider vinegar
1 teaspoon sea salt
16 cups water

Per Serving (1 cup): Calories: 54; Total fat: 3g; Total carbs: 1g; Fiber: <1g' Net carbs: 1g; Protein: 4g; Macronutrients: Fat: 50%; Protein: 30%; Carbs: 20%

1. Preheat the oven to 400°F. Line a baking sheet with parchment paper.
2. Rub the chicken carcasses with the tomato paste and put them on the prepared baking sheet. Roast for 20 minutes.
3. Pick up the parchment paper with the bones and pour the bones and juices into a large stockpot.
4. Add the celery, carrots, onion, vinegar, salt, and water. Stir to combine.
5. Bring the mixture to a boil and then reduce the heat to low and simmer for 12 hours.
6. Let cool for 1 hour and then strain the bones and vegetables out of the broth.
7. Refrigerate for up to 7 days or freeze for up to 3 months.

> **MAKE AHEAD:** You can also make bone broth in a slow cooker. Reduce the water to 12 cups and cook on low for 12 hours.

Fat-Burning Fatty Coffee

SERVES 2 | PREP TIME: 15 MINUTES

Fatty coffee has been a staple in my ketogenic lifestyle since day one. It is rich and filling. Sometimes I can have my fatty coffee in the morning and not be hungry again until dinner. MCT oil has been shown to increase the production of ketones, so this truly is a fat-burning beverage. Two cups of coffee is the magic number for me, as this is the serving size that fits in my Yeti coffee mug.

4 cups brewed coffee
1 tablespoon MCT oil
1 tablespoon
  unsalted butter

Per Serving (2 cups): Calories: 126; Total fat: 13g; Total carbs: 1g; Fiber: 0g' Net carbs: 1g; Protein: 2g; Macronutrients: Fat: 93%; Protein: 6%; Carbs: 1%

1. Preheat a blender by allowing hot water to sit in it while the coffee brews.
2. Pour the coffee, MCT oil, and butter into the blender. Secure the top and hold a few paper towels on top.
3. Start the blender on low and then slowly increase the speed. Blend for 30 to 45 seconds until the mixture is creamy and frothy, like a cappuccino. Serve.

PREPARATION TIP: Two scoops of collagen peptides add creaminess and provide the health benefits of collagen. Make the coffee; then add the collagen and blend for an additional 30 seconds.

Hot Chocolate

SERVES 2 | PREP TIME: 2 MINUTES | COOK TIME: 10 MINUTES

Not to brag, but growing up just outside Hershey, PA, has made me a connoisseur of chocolate. Although you can use heavy cream in place of coconut milk to lower the carb count, I find that coconut milk adds a deeper flavor and texture. To increase the fat-burning power of this hot chocolate, add a tablespoon of MCT oil before blending. Customize with a pinch of cayenne, cinnamon, or whatever you like!

1 cup canned full-fat coconut milk

1 cup unsweetened vanilla almond milk

¼ cup unsweetened cocoa powder

2 tablespoons erythritol

Pinch sea salt

Per Serving (1 cup): Calories: 243; Total fat: 24g; Total carbs: 24g; Fiber: 5g' Sugar alcohols: 12g; Net carbs: 7g; Protein: 4g; Macronutrients: Fat: 81%; Protein: 5%; Carbs: 14%

1. In a medium saucepan over medium heat, whisk together the coconut and almond milks.
2. Raise the heat to medium high and heat just until the milks begin to bubble.
3. Remove from the heat and quickly whisk in the cocoa powder, erythritol, and salt.
4. Pour the mixture into a blender and slowly increase the speed. Blend on high for 1 minute until frothy. Serve.

90-Second Bread

SERVES 1 | PREP TIME: 3 MINUTES | COOK TIME: 1 MINUTE 30 SECONDS

This bread is incredibly versatile, taking on different flavor profiles when various fats and seasonings are used. The base recipe produces a traditional bread flavor that is best used anytime you're craving the comfort of sliced white bread. You can easily add up to 1 tablespoon of erythritol to make this bread sweet.

1 large egg
3 tablespoons almond flour
1 tablespoon melted butter
¼ teaspoon baking powder
Pinch sea salt
Cooking spray

Per Serving (1 bread): Calories: 300; Total fat: 27g; Total carbs: 5g; Fiber: 2g; Net carbs: 3g; Protein: 11g; Macronutrients: Fat: 79%; Protein: 14%; Carbs: 7%

1. In a small bowl, beat the egg with a fork or a whisk.
2. Whisk in the almond flour, butter, baking powder, and salt until completely combined.
3. Spray the inside of a large coffee mug with cooking spray.
4. Pour the mixture into the mug and microwave for 90 seconds.
5. Let the bread cool just slightly and then remove it from the mug. It should slide right out.
6. Slice the bread in half and either enjoy as is, with your preferred toppings, or toasted for some extra crunch.

Essential Fathead Dough

SERVES 8 | PREP TIME: 5 MINUTES | COOK TIME: 1 MINUTE

From pizza to crackers, breads to bagels, sweet rolls, and just about everything in between, fathead dough is an essential keto staple. Two of my favorite ways to use fathead dough are for pizza crust and dinner rolls (especially stuffed with Pulled Pork (page 134). To make this dough dairy-free, use vegan cream cheese.

FOR THE BASE DOUGH

1½ cups shredded mozzarella cheese

¾ cup almond flour

1 ounce full-fat cream cheese

1 large egg, beaten

Per Serving (⅛ recipe): Calories: 150; Total fat: 12g; Total carbs: 3g; Fiber: 1g; Net carbs: 2g; Protein: 7g; Macronutrients: Fat: 72%; Protein: 19%; Carbs: 9%

1. In a large microwave-safe bowl, use a fork to combine the mozzarella and almond flour.
2. Put the cream cheese on top and microwave in 30-second increments, stirring the mixture each time, until the cheeses melt completely, and it begins to look like a dough.
3. Add the egg and mix until completely combined.
4. Use immediately or wrap in plastic and refrigerate for up to 1 week or freeze for up to 1 month. Thaw at room temperature before using.

TO MAKE 1 (10-INCH) PIZZA

1 Essential Fathead Dough recipe

¾ teaspoon dried Italian seasoning

¼ teaspoon garlic powder

Per Serving (1 slice): Calories: 150; Total fat: 12g; Total carbs: 3g; Fiber: 1g; Net carbs: 2g; Protein: 7g; Macronutrients: Fat: 72%; Protein: 19%; Carbs: 9%

1. Preheat the oven to 425°F.
2. Make the basic dough, adding the Italian seasoning and garlic powder in step 1.
3. Roll out the dough between 2 pieces of parchment paper to an ⅛-inch-thick circle.
4. Remove the top layer of paper and poke the dough all over with a fork.
5. Place it on a baking sheet or pizza stone and bake for 7 minutes, until just browned. Flip and bake for another 5 minutes.
6. Remove from the oven and turn the oven to broil.
7. While the oven is heating, top the crust with your desired pizza toppings.
8. Broil for 2 minutes or until the cheese bubbles.

CONTINUED ▶

TO MAKE 8 DINNER ROLLS

1 Essential Fathead
  Dough recipe
1½ tablespoons
  baking powder
1 large egg, beaten
1 tablespoon melted butter

Per Serving (1 roll): Calories: 174; Total fat: 15g; Total carbs: 4g; Fiber: 1g; Net carbs: 3g; Protein: 8g; Macronutrients: Fat: 77%; Protein: 18%; Carbs: 5%

1. Make the basic dough, but add baking powder to the almond flour in step 1 and a second beaten egg in step 3.

2. Form the dough into 8 equal balls. Place the balls in a container and refrigerate for 30 minutes.

3. Preheat the oven to 400°F. Line a baking sheet with parchment paper.

4. Place the dough balls on the prepared baking sheet. Press down on each ball gently to slightly flatten the bottom.

5. Brush the top of each dough ball with the butter.

6. Fill a 9-by-13-inch casserole dish halfway with water. Place the dish on the oven's bottom rack. Place the baking sheet on the middle rack. Bake the rolls for 11 to 15 minutes, until golden. Enjoy immediately.

7. These rolls are best served warm. If you're not planning to serve them right away, refrigerate the dough balls in a container for up to 3 days or freeze for up to 1 month. Thaw in the refrigerator before baking.

Cauliflower Dough

MAKES 8 SLICES | PREP TIME: 50 MINUTES | COOK TIME: 45 MINUTES

I have tried many cauliflower dough recipes, and they have all resulted in a mushy, watery, inedible dish. For a sturdy cauliflower dough that actually has flavor, the secret is precooking the cauliflower rice. It draws out the water and creates a crust that won't break apart while cooking. Roll out the dough evenly so you are not left with parts that are burned and parts that are only half-baked.

2 recipes Caulirice (page 163)
1 large egg, beaten
⅓ cup parmesan cheese
1 teaspoon dried Italian seasoning
½ teaspoon sea salt
½ teaspoon garlic powder
⅛ teaspoon freshly ground black pepper

Per Serving (1 slice): Calories: 56; Total fat: 2g; Total carbs: 7g; Fiber: 2g; Net carbs: 5g; Protein: 4g; Macronutrients: Fat: 32%; Protein: 29%; Carbs: 39%

1. Preheat the oven to 375°F. Line 2 baking sheets with parchment paper. Lay a clean dish towel or 4 sturdy paper towels on top of a large bowl.
2. Spread the caulirice in an even layer on one prepared baking sheet and bake for 15 minutes.
3. Transfer the cooked cauliflower to the bowl and let cool for 15 minutes.
4. Wrap the cooled cauliflower in the dish towel and twist the ends to squeeze out excess water. Continue twisting and squeezing until no liquid remains. (If you are using paper towels, plan to switch them out once they become wet.)
5. In a large bowl, combine the caulirice, egg, parmesan, Italian seasoning, salt, garlic powder, and pepper until thoroughly mixed.
6. Turn the oven up to 450°F.
7. Spread the cauliflower dough evenly on the second prepared baking sheet and bake for 20 minutes.

CONTINUED ▶

8. Remove the crust from the oven, flip, and bake for 5 to 8 more minutes, until the crust is crisp and golden.

9. Refrigerate for up to 3 days or freeze for up to 1 month.

> **FEEDING THE FAMILY:** Make cauliflower dough "breadsticks": Turn the oven to broil. In a small bowl, combine ¾ cup shredded mozzarella cheese, ½ tablespoon olive oil, 2 minced garlic cloves, and ¼ teaspoon red pepper flakes. Spread the mixture evenly on top of the cauliflower crust and broil for 90 seconds. Slice and serve.

Caulirice

MAKES 4 CUPS | PREP TIME: 35 MINUTES

My husband is Latino and grew up eating rice with every meal. When we adopted a keto lifestyle, it was important to find recipes that could mimic his childhood comfort foods. Cauliflower rice for the win! It's white rice's crunchy, low-carb cousin that picks up the flavor of any added spices. If you have a food processor, you can pulse the cauliflower into rice in a snap.

1 small head cauliflower (about 1 pound)
½ teaspoon sea salt

Per Serving (1 cup): Calories: 56; Total fat: 2g; Total carbs: 7g; Fiber: 2g; Net carbs: 5g; Protein: 4g; Macronutrients: Fat: 32%; Protein: 29%; Carbs: 39%

1. Line a baking sheet with paper towels.
2. Remove the green stems and inner core of the cauliflower. Cut the cauliflower head into 4 pieces.
3. Using the large holes of a cheese grater, grate the cauliflower into rice-size pieces.
4. Transfer the caulirice to the prepared baking sheet and season evenly with the salt.
5. Let sit for 15 to 20 minutes for the salt to draw the water out.
6. Place the rice in a clean dish towel or a few sturdy paper towels and squeeze out excess water. Use immediately or refrigerate for up to 3 days.

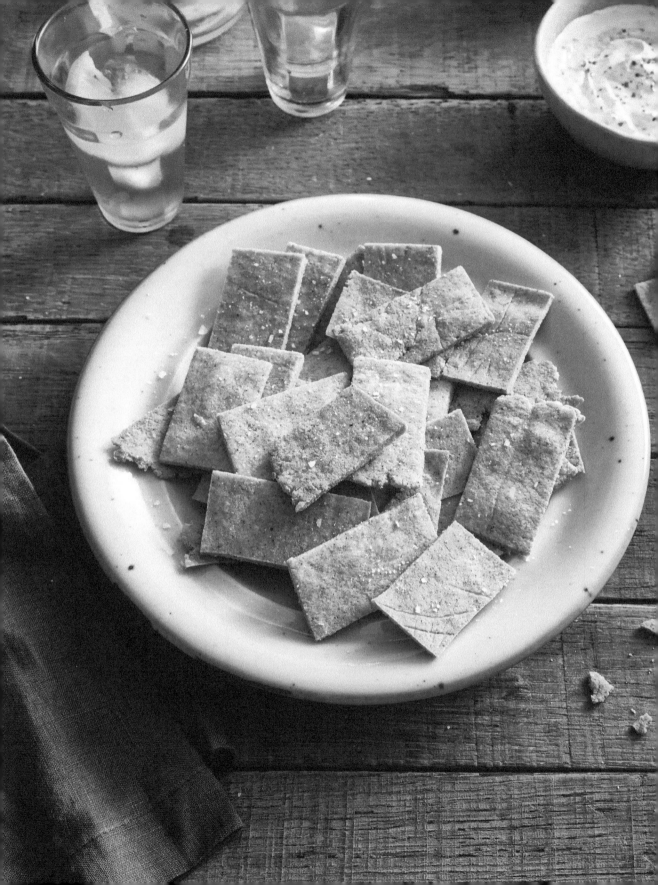

"Cheesy" Tortilla Chips

SERVES 4 | PREP TIME: 25 MINUTES | COOK TIME: 10 MINUTES

You can make tortilla chips out of Essential Fathead Dough (page 159), but they just don't have the same crisp as a regular tortilla chip. Because of the almond flour and egg white—minus the moisture from the cheese—these do! Nutritional yeast, a flaky yellow seasoning used in many vegan recipes to replace dairy, is what gives these chips their cheesy taste.

1 cup almond flour
1 egg white
½ tablespoon avocado oil
1 tablespoon nutritional yeast
1½ teaspoons sea salt, divided
½ teaspoon paprika
½ teaspoon ground cumin
¼ teaspoon garlic powder
⅛ teaspoon chili powder

Per Serving (8 chips): Calories: 187; Total fat: 16g; Total carbs: 7g; Fiber: 4g; Net carbs: 3g; Protein: 8g; Macronutrients: Fat: 77%; Protein: 17%; Carbs: 6%

1. Preheat the oven to 350°F.
2. In a large bowl, combine the almond flour, egg white, oil, nutritional yeast, ½ teaspoon of salt, paprika, cumin, garlic powder, and chili powder. Use your hands to knead the dough until everything is thoroughly combined. Form it into a ball.
3. Place the dough on top of a large piece of parchment paper and top it with another piece of parchment of equal size.
4. Roll the dough out as thin as possible—the thinner the dough, the crispier the chip.
5. Remove the top piece of parchment paper and cut the tortilla dough into 1-inch-by-2-inch strips. Slide the parchment paper with the dough onto a baking sheet.
6. Bake for about 10 minutes, until golden brown.
7. Let cool at room temperature for 10 minutes. Toss the cooled chips with the remaining 1 teaspoon of salt. Serve immediately or store in an airtight container for up to 2 days at room temperature.

Zoodles

MAKES 2 CUPS | PREP TIME: 25 MINUTES

Zucchini noodles—aka zoodles—are a great low-carb pasta replacement and can be served raw or cooked. Drawing out as much water as possible is necessary to ensure the zoodles aren't mushy. Salting the zucchini draws out the moisture. If your zoodles still feel a bit wet, wrap them in a clean dish towel or sturdy paper towels and gently press until most of the water is absorbed.

2 large zucchini, trimmed
½ teaspoon sea salt

Per Serving (½ cup): Calories: 28; Total fat: 1g; Total carbs: 5g; Fiber: 2g; Net carbs: 3g; Protein: 2g; Macronutrients: Fat: 16%; Protein: 18%; Carbs: 66%

1. Place one zucchini at a time in your spiralizer and work it through the spiralizer until it resembles noodles. If you don't have a spiralizer, simply use a vegetable peeler. Peel thin slices until you reach the core. If the slices are too thick for your liking, use a knife to cut them into your desired size.
2. Repeat the process with the second zucchini.
3. A spiralizer produces several very long zucchini noodles, so use a knife or kitchen shears to cut the zoodles into long spaghetti-like pieces.
4. Place the zoodles on a baking sheet and sprinkle with the salt. Let sit for 15 minutes.
5. Pick up the zoodles, shaking off any additional water, and refrigerate for up to 3 days.

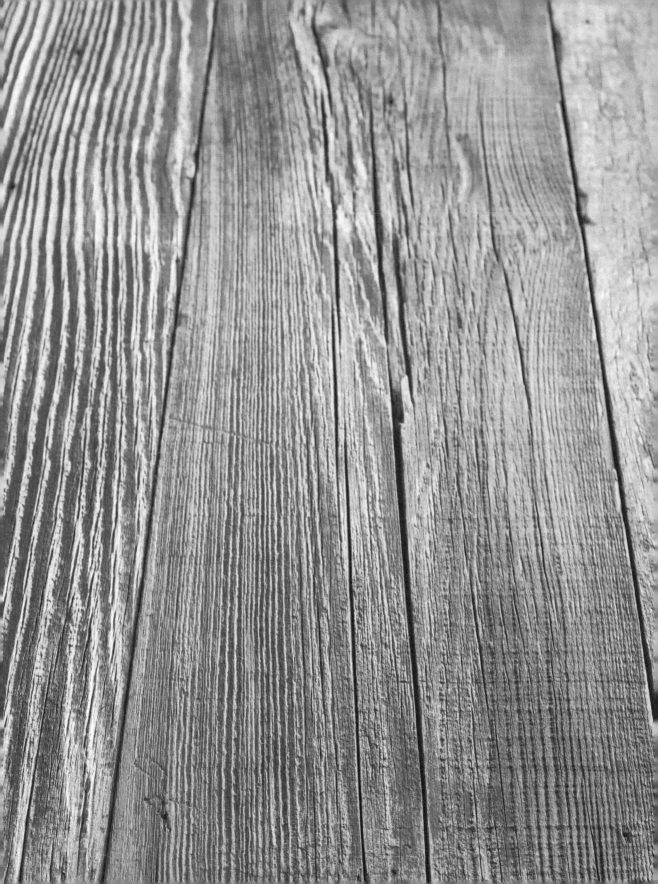

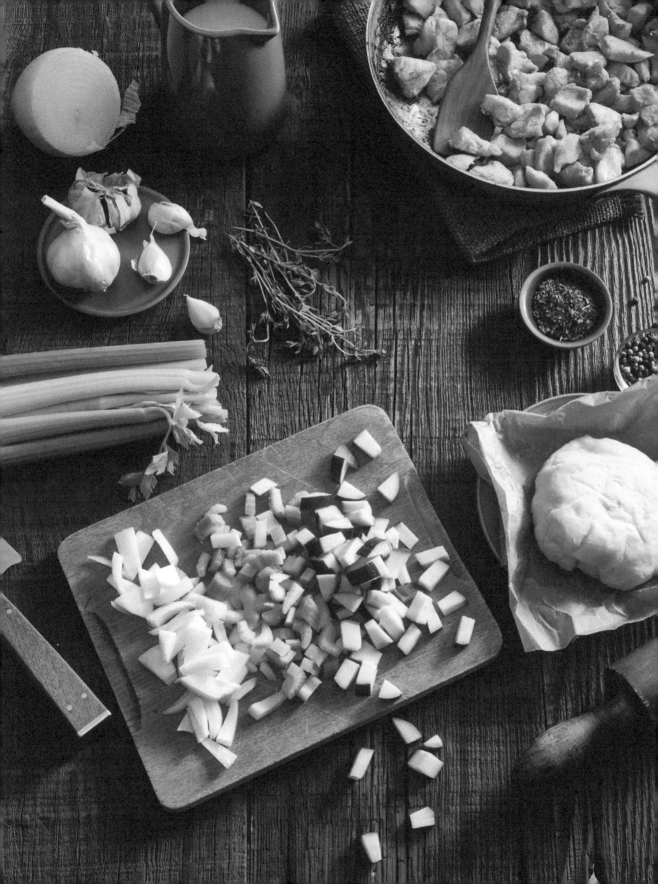

Measurement Conversions

	US STANDARD	US STANDARD (OUNCES)	METRIC (APPROXIMATE)
VOLUME EQUIVALENTS (LIQUID)	2 TABLESPOONS	1 FL. OZ.	30 ML
	¼ CUP	2 FL. OZ.	60 ML
	½ CUP	4 FL. OZ.	120 ML
	1 CUP	8 FL. OZ.	240 ML
	1½ CUPS	12 FL. OZ.	355 ML
	2 CUPS OR 1 PINT	16 FL. OZ.	475 ML
	4 CUPS OR 1 QUART	32 FL. OZ.	1 L
	1 GALLON	128 FL. OZ.	4 L
VOLUME EQUIVALENTS (DRY)	⅛ TEASPOON		0.5 ML
	¼ TEASPOON		1 ML
	½ TEASPOON		2 ML
	¾ TEASPOON		4 ML
	1 TEASPOON		5 ML
	1 TABLESPOON		15 ML
	¼ CUP		59 ML
	⅓ CUP		79 ML
	½ CUP		118 ML
	⅔ CUP		156 ML
	¾ CUP		177 ML
	1 CUP		235 ML
	2 CUPS OR 1 PINT		475 ML
	3 CUPS		700 ML
	4 CUPS OR 1 QUART		1 L
	½ GALLON		2 L
	1 GALLON		4 L
WEIGHT EQUIVALENTS	½ OUNCE		15 G
	1 OUNCE		30 G
	2 OUNCES		60 G
	4 OUNCES		115 G
	8 OUNCES		225 G
	12 OUNCES		340 G
	16 OUNCES OR 1 POUND		455 G

	FAHRENHEIT (F)	CELSIUS (C) (APPROXIMATE)
OVEN TEMPERATURES	250°F	120°C
	300°F	150°C
	325°F	180°C
	375°F	190°C
	400°F	200°C
	425°F	220°C
	450°F	230°C

Resources

CarbManager.com

This app is for those following a low-carb or ketogenic diet and allows you to choose whether you want to track net or total carbs. It is very user-friendly and helps you stay on track with both percentages and colors: green if your macros are good and red if you have gone over. There are both a free and a very low monthly cost versions.

Cronometer.com

Cronometer provides detailed nutrient tracking information and is perfect for someone who wants to look at their macronutrients and their micronutrients. It is possible to track net carbs on this highly detailed app. There is a small monthly fee to use the app on a mobile device.

GetMyMacros.com

Similar to Cronometer, My Macros+ also provides detailed insight on both macro and micronutrient intake. It allows you to enter a variety of nutrition goals and has a database of more than 5 million foods. My Macros+ is $2.99 for lifetime access.

MyFitnessPal.com

MyFitnessPal is a free app with a vast food library. The downside is that the free version is not customizable, and the app does not track net carbs.

Index

M

Macronutrients
general ratios, 3
importance of, 3
tracking, 3, 5
Margarita Pizza Chips, 36
Marinara Sauce, 154
Mascarpone cheese
about, 11
Buttery Caulimash, 58
Cauliflower Mac and Cheese, 59
Hearty Cauliflower Soup, 46–47
MCT oil
about, 11
Fat-Burning Fatty Coffee, 156
Meatballs and Spaghetti, 122–123
Meatloaf, Classic, 114
Meat Marinara Lasagna, 127–128
Mindful eating, 14
Miracle rice
about, 10
Chicken Broccoli Rice Casserole,
104–105
Rice Pudding, 146
Mozzarella cheese
Chicken Parmesan, 97
Essential Fathead Dough, 159–160
Margarita Pizza Chips, 36
Meat Marinara Lasagna, 127–128
Mozzarella Sticks, 37
Sausage-Stuffed Mushrooms, 69
Scalloped Zucchini, 63
Tuna Casserole, 78–79
Turkey Bacon Ranch Casserole, 109
Turkey Tetrazzini, 110
Muffins, Banana Nut, 23
Mug Cake Three Ways, 144
Mushrooms
Beef Stroganoff, 118–119
Chicken Ramen Soup, 43–44
Creamy Green Bean Casserole, 64
Salisbury Steak, 115
Sausage-Stuffed Mushrooms, 69
Tuna Casserole, 78–79
Turkey Tetrazzini, 110

N

Net carbohydrates, 4
90-Second Bread, 158
Noodles. *See also* **Zoodles**
Beef Stroganoff, 118–119
Chicken Ramen Soup, 43–44
shirataki, about, 10
Nuts. *See also* **Almond butter**
almond flour, buying, 10
Banana Nut Muffins, 23
Granola Cereal, 29

O

Oils, smoke points, 9
Olive oil, smoke point, 9
Omelet, Denver, Breakfast Bake, 24
Onion Rings, Bacon-Wrapped, 70
Oven Burgers, 125

P

Pancakes, Ricotta, 21
Parmesan cheese
Brussels Sprouts and Bacon, 65
Cauliflower Dough, 161–162
Chicken Alfredo, 106–107
Chicken Cordon Bleu, 98
Chicken Parmesan, 97
Classic Meatloaf, 114
Creamed Spinach, 72
Creamy Green Bean Casserole, 64
Italian Garden Salad, 51
Meat Marinara Lasagna, 127–128
Mozzarella Sticks, 37
Sausage-Stuffed Mushrooms, 69
Shrimp and Grits, 88
Zucchini Fries, 62
Peppers
Cheesesteak-Stuffed Peppers, 67
Chicken Fajitas, 108
Denver Omelet Breakfast Bake, 24
Italian Garden Salad, 51
jalapeño, handling, 38
Jalapeño Poppers, 38
Shrimp Fried Rice, 85
Sloppy Joes, 129

Acknowledgments

I want to acknowledge and thank everyone who has made this book possible.

Thank you to my parents, husband, and children for your endless support and encouragement.

Thank you to Dr. Josh Axe for introducing me to the ketogenic diet and completely changing the trajectory of my career.

Thank you to my amazing community of Ketogenic Living Certified Coaches who are leading the fat-fueled revolution.

Thank you to the team at Callisto Media for this incredible opportunity, for all your guidance, and for believing in me to create this awesome cookbook.

About the Author

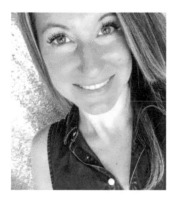

Kate Bay Jaramillo is a ketogenic living expert, wellness mentor, and host of the Straight-Up Wellness podcast. Kate is leading the way in the ketogenic community as the founder of Keto-genic Living 101 and Ketogenic Living 102, creator of the Ketogenic Living Coach Certification, and co-creator of the Keto40.

Kate wholeheartedly believes in the power of a ketogenic lifestyle and is thrilled to have created the first ketogenic coach certification to be approved as a CEU provider for organizations including NASM, AFAA, ISSA, Canfitpro, and CPD. With close to 400 Ketogenic Living Certified Coaches spanning six conti-nents, Kate is thrilled to help spread the fat-fueled health revolution!

When she is not podcasting, mentoring Ketogenic Living Certified Coaches, and creating delicious ketogenic meals, Kate enjoys traveling the world with her husband and four children.